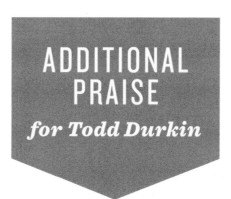

ADDITIONAL PRAISE

for Todd Durkin

"Durkin's passion for fitness is like an adrenaline injection. Although I'm 50 years old, his workouts make me feel like a kid again."

-MILES MCPHERSON, FORMER SAN DIEGO CHARGERS DEFENSIVE BACK AND PASTOR, ROCK CHURCH, SAN DIEGO

"Read this book and let it bring out your best in body, mind, and spirit. Todd knows how to help people be the best they can be."

-KEN BLANCHARD, CO-AUTHOR OF *THE ONE MINUTE MANAGER* AND *LEADING AT A HIGHER LEVEL*

"Durkin is an extraordinary trainer. When TD coaches you, there is no doubt that you will get everything you need and want out of a workout."

-JEFF DILLMAN, HEAD OF PHYSICAL CONDITIONING, IMG PERFORMANCE INSTITUTE

"Todd is a powerhouse of energy, information, and motivation . . . Get ready, because once you pick up this book, your body and life will never be the same!"

-ALI BROWN, FOUNDER AND CEO, ALI INTERNATIONAL AND *ALI MAGAZINE*

THE IMPACT! BODY PLAN

Build New Muscle, Flatten Your Belly & Get Your Mind Right!

Todd Durkin, M.A., C.S.C.S.

with Adam Bornstein and Mike Zimmerman

RODALE®

Men's Health is a registered trademark of Rodale Inc.
IMPACT is a registered trademark of Todd Durkin Enterprises
© 2010 by Todd Durkin

Book design by Mike Smith,
with George Karabotsos, design director of *Men's Health* Books
and Laura White, contributing designer

Photographs by Thomas MacDonald/Rodale Images
Brees and Tomlinson photos © Getty Images
Fascia illustration by Rajeev Doshi/Medi-Mation

Library of Congress Cataloging-in-Publication Data is on file with the publisher.

ISBN-13 978-1-60529-071-3 hardcover

2 4 6 8 10 9 7 5 3 1 hardcover

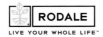

We inspire and enable people to improve their lives and the world around them.

For my mom, Mary Durkin, and my late father, Paul Durkin.
Their unconditional love and unwaivering belief in me
made me the man I am today. They taught me the values of
hard work, commitment, passion, and then some . . .

Memories of my dad inspire me every day.
He gave me the one thing you can't replace or substitute—his time.
He was my biggest fan, always sitting "high up on the
40 yard line," and I'll never forget that.

Mom, you still amaze me!
How you raised the eight of us with such patience, energy, and love,
I'll never know. You are an incredible human being!

And for my beautiful wife, Melanie—an extraordinary person
who makes me feel like the luckiest man alive.
You are my rock, and together we do the most important work of all:
making a family with Luke (7), Brady (5), and McKenna (2).
Thank you for your constant support, love, and belief in me.
I love you!

Acknowledgments

The IMPACT! Body Plan tells part of my personal story and so it has been a pleasure to remember the many people who have touched my life professionally and personally along the path.

First, for my two brothers and five sisters: Stephen, Paul, Patti, Pam, MaryBeth, Judy, and Karen: I always felt so lucky to grow up the youngest of eight. I am blessed to have such loving siblings and wonderful family memories beginning at 13 Edgewood Dr.

I will always be grateful to my mentors:

Coach Wolf: I grew up wanting to be a Green Dragon and play quarterback for the legendary Coach Wolf and powerhouse football at Brick High School in New Jersey. He taught me about life and how to be a man. Wayne Cotton: There are people who come into your life at just the right time. A successful businessman and full of life wisdom, Wayne came into my life just before the opening of Fitness Quest 10. He helped me in more ways than he will ever know and is still a trusted friend and confidant. Tom House: Tom opened my mind on how to train and challenged me to think outside the box. The way I structure my workouts and programs is strongly rooted in his influence.

Patti Durkin: My big sister who told me to always follow my heart, trust my gut, and chase my wildest dreams. It remains some of the best advice I ever received!

Special thanks to the many others who have had IMPACT on my life and professional development: Coach John Sauer (head strength and conditioning coach at The College of William & Mary); Dr. Bruce Costello, Michael and Jena King, Dub and Audrey Leigh, Ali Brown, Chris Poirier and the Perform Better team, Mike Boyle, Thomas Plummer, Gray Cook, and Alwyn Cosgrove.

A huge thank-you to Kevin Plank and the entire Under Armour Team. Kevin taught me that one of the keys to success is surrounding yourself with a great team and great people. I am extremely fortunate to be a part of your team at Under Armour.

To my Fitness Quest 10 Team: You are All-Stars! Thank you Julie, Brett, Ryan R., Ryan B., Chelsey M., Kyle, Doug, Amelia, Karen, Devon, Sammy, Stephanie, Karim, Janet, Anna, Jeff, Chelsea E., Craig, Meg, Matt, Sharon, Mara, Cara, Pat, Chris J., Kim, Megan, Marilou, Linn, Shane, Jenny, Heather, Dr. Kahl, Dr. Jenn, and the wonderful team at Water & Sports Physical Therapy. To the members of the TD Mastermind Group— your drive and desire for excellence in the fitness industry is inspiring! And to all our Fitness Quest 10 clients who have supported our team and me over the past 10 years—I have learned so much from you. Thank you.

To LaDanian Tomlinson and Drew Brees, the first two professional athletes who chose to train with me so many years ago. What an awesome ride it has been to work with each of you. Thank you for entrusting me with your physical conditioning—your most critical asset. You are true champions in all that you do. I have always been inspired by your hard work and dedication and feel blessed to count you as friends.

Writing this book was a labor of love and a lot of hard work! Many thanks go to the IMPACT writing team: Mike Zimmerman and Adam Bornstein. You guys are amazing. I've had the desire to write this book for years, and you helped make it a reality. You showed me what's possible with hard work, a driving conviction, and the right team. Thanks go to George Karabotsos, Mike Smith, Erin Williams, Beth Bazar, Hope Clarke, and Laura White, whose design and editing talents will be appreciated by readers. To all of you: We did it, baby!

And Mary McKay: You are a Godsend. Always there with your support, your writing and editing skills, and your "voice." Thank you so much.

Thanks to Chris Stuart, who represents me so well in so many endeavors. It's great to know you've got my back.

My sincere thanks go to the executive and editorial teams at Rodale, especially Dave Zinczenko, Steve Perrine, and Debbie McHugh, who gave me the opportunity to write this book. What an awesome experience it has been to work with you and your team.

Thank you all from the bottom of my heart!

Contents

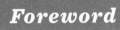

Foreword

QUARTERBACK
DREW BREES
NEW ORLEANS SAINTS

SUPER BOWL XLIV
MVP

NFL Offensive Player
of the Year 2008

Walter Payton NFL Man
of the Year 2006

In order to accomplish something great,

you need people around you who believe in you and instill the
confidence that anything is possible. Todd Durkin is one of those
people for me. Through hard work, discipline, and perseverance,
he helped me realize one of my dreams: winning a Super Bowl.
I remember inviting Todd to Miami for Super Bowl XLIV. I have
trained with him for most of my NFL career, and it was important
to me that he be there to share in this moment. Sure enough,
we won the game, and afterward I remember meeting him at the
team hotel with a big embrace, saying, "We did it, brother. I told you
we would do it." An amazing moment. But few people could
realize how hard Todd and I had both worked to get there because
just 4 years earlier, I couldn't throw a football even 10 yards.

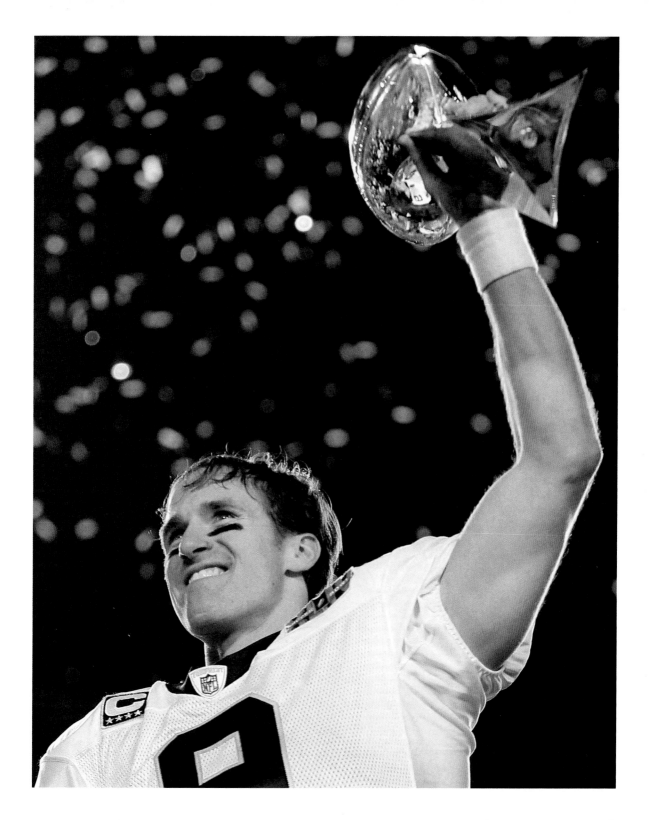

As quarterback of the San Diego Chargers, during the last game of the 2005 season on New Year's Eve, I suffered a devastating injury to my throwing shoulder. Basically it was ripped out of the socket: a 360-degree labrum tear and torn rotator cuff. I had major surgery and a lot of people weren't sure that I would come back from it.

But I knew.

You see, I worked with Todd extensively during my rehab. He never gave up hope. In fact, there was no doubt in his mind that I would come back stronger than ever before. He believed in me, and we pushed our way through together. Training with TD helped fuel a furious comeback.

Two months after surgery, in May 2006, I was picked up by Head Coach Sean Payton and the New Orleans Saints. Eight months later, with my rehab complete, I headed into the 2006 season as their starting quarterback. We had a great year, making it to the NFC Championship game. I was named NFL Man of the Year along with my training partner LaDainian Tomlinson, and was runner-up for NFL MVP to him as well. From a low point early in the year of being without a team, without a job, and possibly looking at the end of my career, to being honored like this was like traveling to the moon and back. A truly magical season.

And then, in 2010: a Super Bowl ring.

Bottom line, TD is one of the main reasons I belonged in that Super Bowl. His commitment to me as one of his athletes has always brought out my best. He is a true champion in every sense of the word. And he always has a plan and a purpose for how he will help you reach your goals.

Even as far back as 2004 when I first walked into Fitness Quest 10 in San Diego to see Todd, I knew something was different. I came to him looking for an edge in my training. Immediately Todd identified my weaknesses by methodically running me through a barrage of exercises. He tested me to see where improvements needed to be made and how hard I was willing to work to remedy them. It was amazing how lacking I was in many areas. I never expected that, and it was just one of many "light bulb" moments I had training with TD. You'll have them, too.

Training with Todd is a lesson in how to exceed your perceived limits. There are times when you feel like you can't do another rep but he finds a way to get it out of you. He breeds competition into the workouts. We push each other and compete against our training partners constantly. This helps us to build tremendous mental and physical toughness, and our confidence soars as we witness the results. This is one thing you'll see as you read his book: TD is a master of the intangibles like motivation and mindset. You can't buy this kind of mental toughness. But you train for it, just like you train your body. And Todd does both better than anyone I've ever met.

Todd is also cutting-edge and he makes you feel like you are on the cutting-edge, too. He constantly brings creative ideas and new and improved movements to my workouts, all with the purpose of making me better. And they work. I feel the improvement and watch it translate to the field.

Todd's energy and enthusiasm are infectious, and you'll feel that as you read his book. When you are around someone who is doing what they love to do and are meant to do, that makes a very strong impact on you. Todd is always thinking about and serving others. He genuinely cares about his clients, not just as athletes but as people. He wants us to feel and be our best in every aspect of life. So it's not just workouts, never just the exercises. He covers every possible edge I can gain from the right diet, sleep habits, recovery, and position-specific training philosophy.

This book gives you the same program Todd and I do together during my off-season. I'm glad he's finally put it all down on paper so other people can benefit. Todd has been a huge part of my success on the football field. He is the best at what he does and is a great example for young athletes and young trainers because he does it right. Stay humble, stay hungry . . . as TD always says.

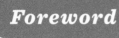

RUNNING BACK
LADAINIAN TOMLINSON
NEW YORK JETS

/ NFL MOST
VALUABLE
PLAYER 2006

When I was a kid, I was a big Walter Payton fan. He was the reason I wanted

to play football. One time I saw him on TV running sprints up a hill
that was outside of Chicago. Later, when I was going into my senior
year of high school, I knew I'd have an opportunity to play running
back. So I figured if it works for Walter, it works for me: I ran hills
all year. After basketball practice, I'd go to the hill. After track
practice, I'd go to the hill. That was a turning point for me. Ever
since high school, I've had a hill, even if I had to have one built.

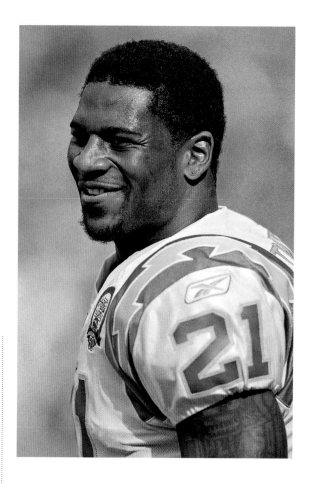

Now, for the past 7 years, before I go to the hill, I go to Todd Durkin. It's no exaggeration to say that TD has been as important to my success as any hill I've run. It comes down to three things:

MOTIVATION: Todd finds a way to motivate everyone he works with. I know it's easy to say that about people—Oh, so-and-so is a great motivator. But in TD's case it's a little bit different. He has this gift for figuring out what will motivate a certain person, like me or you. He trains all kinds of athletes: football players, baseball players, mixed martial arts fighters, as well as executives, housewives, and retired folks. I see them all in his gym and train right next to them. Each person has a different dynamic with Todd, you know? For me, we clicked because I know TD played the game. I know he understands certain things about football that the average trainer may not know if he didn't play. You'll see in this book that he'll connect with you no matter who you are.

ACCOUNTABILITY: This is serious. TD brings the challenge—on the athletic side, sure, but more importantly, with your own goals. He'll ask you, "What's your goal? What do you want to achieve?" And you tell him, thinking that it sounds good. And then he holds you accountable to it. He drives you toward your goal. And he won't stop. He won't let you fall short. In fact, he makes you want not to fall short. That's what's so special.

KNOW-HOW: TD is an encyclopedia. When I first started training with him, he watched me do some things and he gives me this look, and then asks, "LT, do you cut off your right leg more than your left?" And I realized that, yeah, I had a tendency to make a move off the right leg because I was more comfortable doing it. And he said, "Well, there's an imbalance in your left leg, and it's time to work on that." He spotted this before he ever looked at film of me. He pays attention and finds the things you need to work on. That comes from experience and knowledge. That goes beyond what happens in the gym. Todd takes this stuff home. He studies. That's what makes him great.

I like to compare our relationship to a boxer and his trainer. Boxers sometimes only know one thing: training. They don't necessarily know what to do to train. All they know is that they do whatever the trainer says. The trainer sees what the boxer can't see. The trainer understands things the boxer doesn't understand. In that regard, Todd has always told me, especially as I've gotten older, we need to do more of this, less of that to maintain your edge, your high level of performance. And I do it, because I trust him. Why do I trust him?

When I first started with him, I didn't understand exactly what we were doing. But I could feel myself getting better. My balance was better. My core was stronger. Before I met Todd, I'd always been strong everywhere else, but my core was my weakest link. He introduced me to my core. And I started to see things change. I remember after working with him for a while that when I hit the field, my movements were so effortless. It was like people couldn't catch me. I was untouchable. It was amazing. That's when I was sold on TD's program.

But here's the biggest thing: I know that because of these workouts, when there are 5 minutes left in the fourth quarter of a close game, I never have to ask myself, "Can I get this done?" Negative thoughts never enter my brain. Knowing you have that level of fitness, because you've worked for it and proved it, gets right in your brain at the toughest times. You're gonna get it done. You're gonna find a way.

That's Todd Durkin's magic.

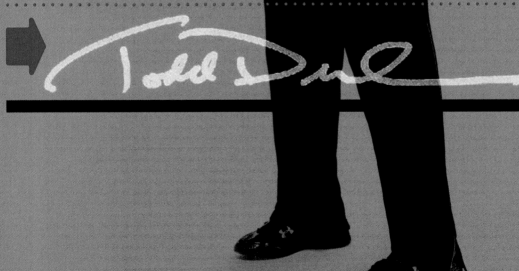

1
MY STORY IS YOUR STORY

I lay on my back staring up

at the pristine blue sky of Aix-en-Provence, the kind of spring day in southern France that dreams are made of . . . and my dream was dead. I couldn't move my legs. I blinked, disoriented, felt my heart in my ears, sounds around me echoing inside my helmet, coaches and trainers staring down at me, my brain sending signals to move my legs, move anything. Nothing worked. I was hurt bad and I knew it. Everything beautiful about where I was—25 years old, playing American-style pro football in the south of France, dreaming of getting to the NFL—gone.

A few seconds earlier, it was third and long, the center snapped me the ball, and I was rolling right of the pocket, the number 10 on my jersey, looking downfield for a receiver. The coverage was tight; it wasn't happening. I tucked the ball and ran it myself, pounding for yardage. Four yards, 5, and more. There, first down, baby, I made the first down. I could sense the defense closing in. Didn't know how many, but it wasn't time to get greedy.

I hook-slid like all quarterbacks are trained to do after they're finished running the ball, the foot-first slide move that guarantees my safety, signals to the defense that I'm officially down and they can't hit me.

And then: **BOOM! . . . IMPACT.**

Two linebackers crushed me at full speed, helmets into my back. And my entire life stopped dead.

That day changed everything for me. And now I hope this day—the day you started reading this book—will change everything for you. Take a look in the mirror. Are you where you want to be? Are you fit? Are you happy? Are you satisfied with your story?

More likely, if you've come to this book, something may be missing. Maybe you're like I was: struggling in a body that hurts and is always in pain. Or maybe you are overweight, or you don't feel great, or your energy is not where you want it to be. You probably have dreams—but you're no longer sure how to achieve them. You're broken. I know how this feels.

Or maybe you've just hit a barrier, reached a plateau, and need help getting to the next level. You're putting in the time but not making progress. Your routines are stagnant. You're bored. You're searching.

Or, possibly, you're like many of my clients. You're ambitious and competitive. You're fit and healthy. You do work hard. Every day. And if there's more, you want it. You love challenges. You strive to be your best. You will do what it takes to achieve your best. I know how this feels, too.

Everyone who comes to see me asks me to help them, to change them. Some are broken and "paralyzed." Some are stuck and bored. Some are just hungry for more. You know your story best.

In 1996 in southern France before I took that hit, I felt unstoppable. Until I wasn't. It's no sin to take a hit. (Or to feel stuck. Or to want it all.) You rarely see the hit coming, especially the cheap shots. But what do you do with the hit? That's the test. Hits can be fate. Hits can be fuel. Hits can deliver a game-changing IMPACT that transforms your entire life.

That's what happened to me. Ever since I took that hit, I've been on a wild ride to cure my own pain, help other people cure theirs, and lead as many as I can into peak physical conditioning—which is the secret to achieving a world-class life.

Of course, I didn't know that at the time. . . .

Once they helped me off the field, I realized that I wasn't paralyzed—in the traditional sense, anyway. I'd had five concussions in my football career, endless pains, strains, and sprains. But this scared me. This was different. My back pain was so excruciating, so all-consuming, that I could hardly move. I started seeing the downside of where I was, what I was doing. I realized the south of France was thousands of miles away from everyone who mattered to me. My French doctors spoke little English. And when the initial diagnosis was translated for me? "Back strain." I'm thinking, "Are you kidding me?"

Still, I refused to be done. My instinct was to battle through. They shot me up with painkillers,

COMMITMENT + CONNECTING +

and I played the next game—which in retrospect was one of the stupidest things I've ever done. I played well. No one touched me. It was my birthday weekend. My mom and sister Patti had come to town, and after the game we went out to dinner. That's when the painkillers wore off. I've never felt agony like that before. I literally felt paralyzed. The pain was excruciating, and the fear of the unknown was debilitating. This time it put me in the hospital. I needed help walking to the bathroom. Feeding myself. I was terrified. What was next? What did the future hold?

Y ou have a story like mine. It may not involve sports or an injury. But you're here for a reason. You've taken a hit. You want fresh movement. New energy. Change. Transformation. I found a way back, and now I'm going to show you that path. You can create a life of freedom based on health and conditioning. It all starts there. I believe physical conditioning is at the center of it all. When you combine commitment to a program and to yourself, conditioning of your body/mind/spirit, and connecting in positive ways with great people, you get creation. When you're in the best shape of your life, eating right, sleeping well, and feeling great, that's when you achieve an energy shift. Your energy can be directed toward creation. And you can create whatever you want.

But this is very important: *Do not ask me to fix you.* I won't. I can't. Because one thing I know for certain is that action is the key to getting to the next level in your life. And you need to be the one who takes the action. I can coach you and give you the program, but you need to make the commitment to get better.

One of my mantras—and you'll see in this book that I have a few—is "Ready, fire, aim." Most of us live by the mantra "Ready, aim . . . aim . . . aim." And we never fire. You say you want to start an exercise program, but you never do; you say you want to hire a trainer to get you into shape, but you never do; you say you're going to get a better job, but you never do; you say you're going back to school, reconnecting with the people you love, traveling to a long-dreamed-of locale.

You never do.

That's why I live by "Ready, fire, aim"—it forces me to take action even when I feel fear, or hesitation, or uncertainty. This program is all about action. I'll give you the game plan. You take the action. I'll motivate you. Inspire you. Coach you. I'll also hold you accountable. (You'll see how in Chapter 3.) But, folks, have no illusions. You have to take action. You need to be there for yourself. You need *you.*

I believe all of us have the potential to be "world class" in our lives—whether as a parent, in our career, as an athlete, or whatever our dreams were as a child. But somewhere along the line, many

CONDITIONING = Creation

of us get sidetracked by limiting beliefs that rob us of our potential. We hesitate. We stop. I'm here to say that now is the time to shoot for best in class. This program shows you what it takes to be world class with your conditioning, the root of greatness in all areas of your life.

W hen the doctors finally did an MRI on my back, the verdict was in: My football career was over. I had three herniated disks, spinal stenosis, and advanced degenerative back disease. "You have zee back of a 75-year-old man," a doctor told me, French accent and all. And so I was told I would need surgery. And I thought, "But not in France. Not now. I'll deal with the pain until I can get home." The problem was I couldn't even sit up, let alone ride in a plane for 9 hours back to the States.

I spent the next month at my small studio in France, most of the time in bed, on crutches, still needing help doing the simplest little things. A nurse stopped by twice a day to shoot me up with painkillers and anti-inflammatories. It was a very introspective time in my life. I knew I had to move on to the next chapter . . . but to what? All I ever wanted to do was play pro football, make my family proud, make my friends back in Brick, New Jersey, proud. I believed, truly believed, that I could play in the NFL. And now I was finished.

I had options, though I didn't care. I'd already completed my degree in kinesiology from The College of William & Mary, already had my massage therapy certificate, already had plenty of education and skill to fall back on. But none of this occurred to me then, because I wanted to play in the NFL.

Meanwhile, the physical therapist and osteopath I worked with every day in France showed me what they were doing for me and why—the therapy, the acupuncture, the energy work, everything. You

"Do or do not. There is no try."

— YODA

name the modality, I was doing it. And when I was finished being treated, I would just hang out in the clinic and watch them treat people. I wasn't totally aware of it, but my new journey had begun: healing. I learned as much from them as I had in school. My back pain had led me to and was teaching me about all the treatments that I would eventually use or recommend to my own clients someday.

After 3 months, I was finally able to fly home to New Jersey. I spent a lot of time hanging around my sister Patti's day spa, Therapeutic Touch, in Bay Head. I was able to work on my back and find a lot of solitude. I continued to refuse surgery. One day I was sitting on the porch of the spa, and a woman came out—one of my sister's clients, I guessed—and she said, "I heard you're Patti's brother and that you just finished playing football in France. She said you were one heck of an athlete."

I chuckled. "Yeah, I was an athlete. Still an athlete in mind, I guess. I'm working on my back, but . . . yeah."

"Do you do personal training?" she asked. "Massage therapy?"

I smiled and said, "Sure do!" even though I didn't have much experience at that point.

"Do you do in-home work?"

I smiled wider. "Let me check my schedule. . . . Absolutely!"

She explained that her husband was a former athlete with a bad back and he needed help with it. "I'd love for you to meet with him."

Now I didn't know who this woman was, or her husband. So she calls me and sets up an appointment. The address: 1 Mount Street in Bay Head. And I'm thinking, "1 Mount Street, 1 Mount Street . . . wait a second. That's the big mansion on the beach."

I called Patti and asked her who that woman was. "That's Jena King," she said. "Michael King's wife."

You may not know who Michael King is, but you know his work. He's the CEO of King World Productions, which produced *Oprah, Wheel of Fortune, Jeopardy!* and a lot more. His dad created *The Little Rascals.*

Michael and I hit it off. He's a stocky Irishman with red hair and is just . . . intense. You could tell by his drive why he was so successful. He was charismatic and energetic, and loved sports. He wanted me to do massage and exercise therapy and personal training for his back—which was comical, a guy with a bad back hiring a guy with a bad back to fix him. But Michael took me under his wing. I started learning what it meant to be an entrepreneur, a businessman. It was a different world—he had executives come down to the beach house from New York City all summer. On the 4th of July, the Grucci family shot fireworks off Michael and Jena's balcony. And there I am on the deck doing massage therapy on all these people, looking out at the ocean, thinking, "Man, 3 months ago I'm flat on my back on a French football field. Now I'm here. How does this all fit in? How could this be the path God intended for me?"

I couldn't figure it out. But not long after this, Michael put me to the test. As that summer played

out, I had applied to Auburn University for graduate school. I was accepted, I had a condo picked out, I had a teaching assistantship lined up. A legitimate "next chapter" for me. And Michael tosses a wrench into the works: "Why don't you come out to L.A. with me?"

I turned him down. After all, I had my next chapter ready to go. I told him my goal was to get my graduate degree. Michael isn't one to take no for an answer, however. He kept trying to tempt me to go to L.A. The days ticked down to my departure for Auburn. And he finally said to me, "Todd, listen. You want to be in the health and fitness field. You're good. Come to the West Coast with me and do it out there. I know everyone in the entertainment business. I can help you get started. Everything migrates from west to east, so you'll be able to build and expand what you do as much as you want. You can go to grad school anytime. You want to go later, I'll even pay for it. But I need you in L.A. This is your ticket."

I couldn't refuse.

L.A. was crazy. Michael's Brentwood house was being built, so he rented Sting's beach house in Malibu. I stayed in the guesthouse. Tom Hanks lived on one side, Rob Reiner on the other. On Halloween, Hanks brought his kids by to trick-or-treat. I answered the door, and while I was handing out candy, I said, "You look like Tom Hanks."

"Great costume, huh?" he said.

It was a strange time for me. Jersey boy on the West Coast. Working for Michael. I was exposed to a special mindset, up close and personal with one of the best-of-the-best entrepreneurs. Michael's vision, fearlessness, and larger-than-life living. I loved that attitude. But in a way, this life didn't feel real for me. Was the boy from Jersey feeling out of place in L.A.? Or was it something else? Something was missing.

I was about to meet someone else who would IMPACT my life in yet another powerful way.

By the time I was entrenched in L.A., I had been on Vicodin for 9 months for my back. The pills were my constant companion, my crutch, my secret to day-to-day functioning. If I missed a pill, I couldn't move. My back wasn't healed. I was hooked.

My sister Patti had heard of this man named Dub Leigh and thought that maybe he could help me with my back issues. Based in Hawaii, Dub was teaching a form of bodywork called Zen Bodytherapy in L.A. during late 1996 through early '97. He delivered the program in a series of 10 specific, exacting sessions. Patti told me that if I did it, she would do it as well, flying out from Jersey for 5 weekends, two sessions per weekend, Saturday and Sunday. So I said, "I'll do it," not really understanding who Dub was or what I was signing up for.

Eighty-year-old Dub was an unassuming guy; he always dressed in khakis and a polo shirt, but he was a bit brash. He referred to people by using funny, whimsical nicknames, like "ding-dong" or "dummy." But you also could tell he was like a big teddy bear. His vast knowledge and program were a little intimidating. That first workshop started with me sitting *zazen* for 1 hour. Zazen is a very strict form of meditation in which you don't move. At all. You cross your legs, sit upright, and cross your hands right below your belly button, and you gaze out to the horizon, eyes open the whole time, and maintain posture by trying to extend the top of your head to the sky. You do this in a circle, facing everyone else in the workshop. If you move, Dub hits this big gong, which reminds you to remain silent without moving. If you sweat, don't wipe it. Itch? Don't scratch it. It was a special form of torture for me.

So I'm sitting there, my back screaming, my muscles quaking, thinking, "I gotta quit. I can't do this. This is ridiculous."

I never quit anything. So I learned something

THE IMPACT BODY PLAN *Promise*

THIS PROGRAM IS designed to transform your overall health: body, mind, and spirit. By committing to this approach, you'll improve at least 10 different aspects of your health and fitness, including:

Physical performance in both everyday activities and the sports you love

Overall strength

Fast-twitch muscle fiber development

Chronic pain in your back, knees, and other common areas

Coordination

Metabolism

Stress levels

Blood pressure and heart rate

Fat loss and inches lost

Mindset

that day: If you don't like something, you probably need it.

Over the course of his life, Dub Leigh had lived with three of the biggest pioneers in Eastern healing and massage/bodywork: Ida Rolf (Rolfing), Moshe Feldenkrais (Feldenkrais), and Tanouye Roshi (energy work). Dub believed that when you were energetically balanced, serene, and in touch with your inner self, healing could begin. Thus the zazen challenge that I was failing. Serene? I had a lump of anxiety in my belly. How could I possibly finish this?

They gonged me several times. They propped me up with pillows under my hips to help me get more comfortable. And eventually I made the hour. This was just the first session. Every one of the 10 sessions would begin with an hour sitting zazen.

What I came to realize is that sitting zazen is not only an important part of this work, it's an important part of the day, every day, to help with your own energy balance and healing. It is stillness. This isn't some Eastern mumbo jumbo. It's real. It works. Even now, the days I sit zazen, I feel more in balance, and my hips feel better, and my back feels great. The bad days can't touch me.

When Dub started working on my body, I would experience the most profound lesson of my life. Sessions four, five, and six of Zen Bodytherapy focus on your hips. Specifically, your hip rotators and psoas (pronounced so-az) muscles, which are your deep hip flexors—a pair of long muscles about the size of your forearms that are located on the anterior part of your spine and run down through your pelvis to the tops of your femurs. They contribute to the flexion and internal rotation of the hip joints. Your hip rotators are your glutes and lateral hip muscles, which often get tight when back pain is present. (Or are they tight and then back pain appears? Hmmm . . . Keep reading.)

By this time, I had begun graduate classes at San Diego State University, so I was commuting back and forth between San Diego and L.A. The driving killed my back. I still leaned hard on the Vicodin to get me through each day. Without it, I was crippled.

So Dub started in with the psoas muscles and hip rotators, an area of the body where most people are very, very tight. As he worked on me, it was the weirdest thing. He started coughing. And he said, "Ugh, you're toxic."

I'm thinking, "What the heck's this guy talking about, toxic? I'm one of the healthiest people I know."

He dug into my hip rotators with his elbows. His large-framed Okinawan wife, Audrey, held me down. Man, his elbow felt like a sword sticking through my hips and glutes. "What did you do to yourself, ding-dong?" Dub asked. "You are one messed-up guy. Your pain isn't coming from your back. It's originating from your tight hips. When we release your hips, we will release your life."

He worked on me for about an hour that day. He continued to cough. Continued telling me I was toxic. And I'm thinking, "How does he sense this?" Now, in retrospect, I believe he was a genuine healer, so in tune with my body.

That night I drove down the 405 freeway back to San Diego. Out of nowhere I felt gurgling in my stomach, my head started to pound, and a wave of something hit me hard, like the worst and fastest stomach bug in history. I pulled over and puked, just emptied myself out. I felt diarrhea coming on. Cold sweats. Just massively sick. But the weird thing . . . I wasn't sick. The vomit left a weird, mysterious taste in my mouth. Metallic.

When I got home that night, same thing. Sick again, with this weird taste in my mouth. The next day, in biomechanics class, it hit me again. I ran outside and puked on the lawn, and this time it was like puking pure metal. Now I'm freaked out. I called Dub and asked him, "What is this? I'm not sick, but I'm puking every few hours. And it tastes like metal!"

"Todd" (I think it was the first time he used my name), he said, "you're detoxing 9 months of Vicodin and everything else wrong in your system. This is part of the healing process. I will see you up here this weekend for the rest of your healing." And he hung up on me.

So I went. Session four. Session five. Session six. Three weeks later, and lots of puking and diarrhea along the way, the hip work finally ended, and so did my back pain. I was pain free. I haven't touched Vicodin—or needed to—since.

What's your story like? I'll bet that in its own way, your story hits all the same mileposts as mine: You're working on your dream when life throws a curve. You go down, and before you know it, you're gazing up at a blue sky, looking for answers, wondering what happened. How do you rise up and move again? How do you transform yourself?

Read this book.

My experience proved to me that there are many avenues to healing, more than we know. We're used to the pills, the scalpels, the hospitals. And bless those surgeons when we do need them. Stated simply, I believe that so much healing can happen if we just open our minds and discover the true root of our problems.

The IMPACT program is based on everything I've learned through all my experiences: education, conditioning, professional sports, pain, Vicodin dependency, Western and Eastern healing. Dub Leigh didn't just treat me. He trained me. I finished the certification program for his method of bodywork—where I learned about little-known yet crucial keys to wellness like the psoas and fascia, an exotic-sounding system of the body that I'll teach you all about in the coming chapters.

Adding Dub's wisdom to my own skill set helped push me toward my dream of helping people achieve wellness. Michael King's entrepreneurial drive inspired me as well. I eventually turned down a teaching and strength-and-conditioning coaching position at an L.A. college so I could open a small personal training studio in San Diego in the year 2000. Fitness Quest 10 was born upon a dream, and this allowed me to combine the best of the "Western" fitness and sports conditioning world with the best of the "Eastern" healing world. I turned down salary, benefits, stability, and potential tenure to become an entrepreneur. I took action. Ready, fire, aim. No money, no clients, no business plan. No problem!

As I write this, Fitness Quest 10 has grown to be a world-class center that combines personal training, massage and bodywork, sports performance training, Pilates, yoga, nutrition, physical therapy, chiropractic, life coaching, and more. My team and I have had the opportunity to help thousands of people looking for an edge in their health and performance.

Today, I train some of the best professional athletes in the world right alongside some of the most dedicated average Joes and Janes striving to be great in their own fitness and life performance. (More than 50 percent of our clients are women.) Now I'm taking the next step in my dream—and you hold it in your hand. This book and the program within will help you transform your entire life.

I call this program IMPACT: a comprehensive, 10-week body/mind fitness plan that will not just build muscle and melt fat—which is what everyone wants—but will also turn your body into a high-performance machine. You'll look and feel better, of course, but you'll also think better and perform better. I'll work you head to toe, inside and out.

One last thing you need to know before I turn you loose on this program: The number 10 has special significance to me. It's stamped all over my life. You'll see it come up again and again in this book. Ten represents world class. The ultimate effort. We constantly rate things on a scale of 1 to 10. Ten is the best. At Fitness Quest 10, everyone who works there is given a credo card describing what 10 means for us: "10 represents a perfect number. This is the quest for success in our lives and our clients' lives. If you put a 10 into everything you do, you'll get a 10 out of it." And that is the source of another saying you'll encounter in this book: 10 in—10 out.

It takes a 10 effort to get anywhere in every aspect of your life: physically, mentally, emotionally, spiritually, nutritionally, you name it. That's the formula. You can't say, "I want to lose 20 pounds," and put in a 7 effort. You'll never get there. No more than Drew Brees can say, "I want to win a Super Bowl," and expect to get there on an 8.5 effort level in his training. Drew trains at a 10 effort—and then some—in all his training sessions. And he won the Super Bowl.

10 in—10 out. Do the work and you will get unbelievable results. This is an action-oriented program, and you don't get results just from reading the book. Take action. Fire.

"Nothing happens until something starts moving."

—ALBERT EINSTEIN

"Physical fitness is not only one of the keys to a healthy body. It is the basis of dynamic and creative intellectual activity. The relationship between the soundness of the body and the activities of the mind is subtle and complex. Much is not yet understood. But we do know what the Greeks knew: That intelligence and skill can only function at the peak of their capacity when the body is healthy and strong; that hardy spirits and tough minds usually inhabit sound bodies."
— JOHN F. KENNEDY

2
MY COMMITMENT TO YOU

I designed this book to be a game changer

for fitness, and a life changer for you. If you commit to this 10-week IMPACT program, I promise that your life as you know it will change. Your body will change, of course. But your mind and spirit will change, as well. President Kennedy knew what he was talking about in that quote. Total fitness, the state of being truly fit, must include the mind and spirit as well as the body, or the entire machine will malfunction.

Why? Physical, mental, and spiritual conditioning drives success in every area of your life. You want to change a relationship? Start with your conditioning. You want to change your energy? Start with your conditioning. You want to change your financial status? Start with your conditioning. Everything comes back to that.

If you're thinking, "I'm just here for the workout" or "I want to see what the pros do," that's fine. You will sweat and sweat some more, my friend. I'm going to give you a cutting-edge exercise program built on my personal philosophy that includes the best science, the best equipment, the best techniques. An approach that you will not find in your average gym or workout book. You'll also get a huge bonus: total transformation—true fitness—from the inside out. That's a promise.

You'll achieve this by using the most ingeniously designed exercise machine ever created: your body. You'll be doing things that are years ahead of what everyone else you know is doing. You'll discover what really matters in a great workout program. You'll also discover that you have far more ability than you think. You may not be a professional athlete, or even athletic at all, but you'll see the transformation you've earned from the "10 in—10 out" formula. You will discover a fire within you, a white-hot, metabolism-boosting, body-transforming inferno that you will stoke all by yourself—and it will never go out again.

And that's just the beginning. I've tapped a lifetime of experience and learning to bring together the ultimate fitness toolbox. So if you scoff and ask, "What makes your book so different?" here are a few things to consider.

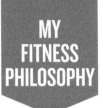

MY FITNESS PHILOSOPHY

YOU'LL READ A lot in this book about what I believe. But as far as my overarching fitness philosophy: It's about results. There is no single utopia for all. Some people need more flexibility and recovery. Some people need more strength work. The purpose of this program is to give you a comprehensive view of what it takes to be the best you can be. The program will get you results no matter where you are physically. Most people's view of "appropriate intensity" is different from my view of appropriate intensity. I believe you train for dynamic movement, not to always lie on a bench and press weights. Training should be multidirectional, multiplanar. I believe in capturing the play element in exercise. I also believe there is an athlete in each of us. My goal is to train that athlete—no matter his or her talent—for peak performance.

1 You'll do the exact same workouts the pro athletes do, and you'll learn their training secrets.

People pay a lot of attention to how many pro athletes I train. You'll see their names and motivational stories throughout the book. They come to me, they trust me, and we work hard together to take their already-elevated games to entirely new levels. But guess what? You will be doing the exact same program that I put the pros through. You will do the exercises that Drew Brees does, that LaDainian Tomlinson does, that Aaron Rodgers does, that players from the Chargers, Saints, Jets, Bears, Packers, Vikings, Falcons, 49ers, Panthers, Rams, Buccaneers, Ravens,

The Motivator /// Whenever you come across something in this book that you don't like, I'll tell you what I tell my athletes: You don't like it because you need to do it. You know how many times I've heard an athlete mutter, "Aw, I hate that drill." That's because they need to do it. Cherry-picking from this book only weakens the overall impact. When you get with a program, get with the whole program, and know you've earned the results.

Padres, Phillies, White Sox, and Rangers do.

Every client who comes through my door at Fitness Quest 10 gets the same treatment, whether they're 70-year-old retirees, fortysomething deconditioned ex-jocks, or high school kids looking for an edge. I've got grandparents who can outwork, outperform, and outlast you. At my place, the average Joes train alongside the pros, literally. Why do I do this? Well, why separate them? They're searching for the same thing.

If you want to be successful at anything, you have to train like a professional athlete. They are some of the best learners and teachers I know. These athletes make a living from their bodies, so when they find something that works or gives them an edge or a breakthrough, they embrace it. Now you get to hear about the unique workout secrets that helped them the most.

2 Workouts will require less time and feel more like play.

We've lost the concept of "playtime" as adults. At Fitness Quest 10, my goal for my clients is to have recess all over again. Like we did when we were kids. Sweat. Smile. Run and play. The average child smiles thousands of times a day. How many times a day do you smile? You probably need to do it more. Research has shown that people who smile more have less incidence of heart attack, stroke, and cancer. The IMPACT program is designed to put a smile on your face. And the workouts are shorter than you imagine. It's a fact that people respond to a positive atmosphere. I run classes where clients joke, laugh, and, most important, play. Even at my 6:30 a.m. class, filled mostly with 50-something professionals, there is nowhere else on Earth they would rather be. We achieve playtime two ways—an ever-changing and challenging workout that is never boring, and a

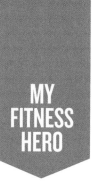

MY FITNESS HERO

WHEN I FIRST opened my facility, Fitness Quest 10, in 2000, an older woman hobbled up my stairs, aching and visibly in pain. Her body was out of balance, and she needed something, anything, to take her pain away. She was 60 years old and an active tennis player but didn't know how to condition her body properly and keep it from constantly breaking down. Now, 10 years later, at the ripe young age of 70, Donna Dickinson is one of the fittest athletes I work with. And that includes all my pro athletes. She practices yoga and breathing work every morning, uses my training program 3 days a week, and plays tennis 5 days a week. Donna adopted the style of training you'll find here—the same one my pros use—and her routine allows her to act decades younger than her age.

"Whether you think you can or think you can't . . . you're right!"

— HENRY FORD

positive mental attitude throughout. How can you not have a positive mental attitude while exercising? You're doing the best thing you can for yourself. Be ecstatic about that. And be thankful that this program is all about time efficiency. There is no reason in the world why you can't get an intense, sweat-soaked, boo-yah-baby total-body workout in 60 minutes or less. It will put a smile on your face every time.

"Go out on a limb. That's where the fruit is."

— WILL ROGERS

3 You will stop getting hurt, and your chronic aches and pains will fade into the past.

You'll discover a new level of flexibility when you learn about and work on your fascia. What is your fascia? To me, the fascia is the most overlooked aspect of any system in our bodies. Fascia is a 3-D, cobweb-like substance that is intertwined around every muscle, tendon, ligament, nerve, and bone in your body. From feet to fingertips, left to right, front to back, we are one big fascial sheath. To give you an idea of what it looks like, the next time you're at the supermarket meat counter, look at the web-like coating on raw, skinless chicken or the silver sinew on a piece of raw filet mignon. That's fascia. Our human fascia is similar. And when your back, hips, knees, neck, or shoulders start to hurt, your fascia gets involved. It tightens. It knots. The body tries to correct itself but can't figure out how, and some areas compensate for others. That brings pain.

One of the easiest ways to illustrate how you can lengthen and loosen your fascia is to roll a tennis ball along the underside of your foot. The pressure from the ball begins to work out the tightness in the fascia. Try it for a few minutes. I guarantee you'll feel a difference. The IMPACT program addresses fascia in all areas of your body.

I am also convinced that besides physical pain being held in the fascia, you can also carry emotional or spiritual trauma in the fascial system. I have had men and women break down and weep on a massage table after I've done fascial work on

---

The Motivator /// Get used to this concept: "And then some." It's the added spice. The heat. It's like turning up the volume. Do your workout, and then some. Commit to this program, and then some. Weight loss, job performance, relationships, parenting? And then some. "And then some" pushes you through limitations. It's your ticket to world-class performance in everything you do. You'll see it often in this book: And then some.

them. They don't cry because it hurts, but because there is a release, and all the junk they've kept stored in their body and in their lives comes out. Very few people know about or target the fascia as an element of fitness. But it's real.

A few years ago I taught at a pitching clinic run by my colleague and friend Tom House. I spoke only on flexibility and fascia to pitchers and pitching coaches. So I gave my spiel: If you took everyone who had recent orthopedic surgery and went back in time to put them on a strict flexibility and fascia-lengthening program—integrating foam rolling, stretching, and bodywork—before they got hurt, half of them would probably never have needed surgery.

When I finished, a hand went up near the back. The man said, "Todd, great job on the talk. My name is Dr. Todd Lanman. I'm the head neurosurgeon at Cedars-Sinai Hospital in L.A."

THE FASCIA

Fascia is the weblike sheath that envelops every muscle, tendon, ligament, nerve, vein, and artery of the body. It supports your organs and joints from head to toe, acts as a shock absorber, and is extremely rich in nerve supply. Your strength, flexibility, and fitness performance depend on its health.

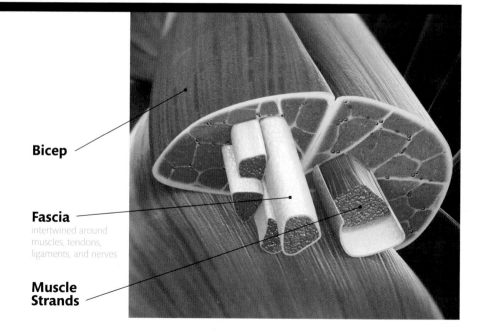

Bicep

Fascia
intertwined around muscles, tendons, ligaments, and nerves

Muscle Strands

I thought, "Oh boy, spine surgeon, here we go; we're gonna have a battle." You have the neurosurgeon on one side, and then you have me, "personal training dude," on the other. And Dr. Lanman said, "You're absolutely right. We can't directly address fascia as physicians. We're not trained for it, and we don't have time to address it. Those 50 percent will never get into a program like you describe, they'll have their surgeries, and we'll probably see them again in 2 years because lifestyle changes were not made and fascia and flexibility were not improved. The fascial restrictions will eventually negatively affect the kinetic chain, and pain will be reproduced." He told the group that fascial work and flexibility work were some of the smartest preventive medicine they could find. And that was a terrific affirmation for me.

My point? You need to address the fascia. And while you can receive hands-on bodywork, you can also do the dynamic warmup portion of my training program. It helps to activate the nervous system and addresses mobility and fascia. Not many people start their workouts this way. And I guarantee this approach will go a long way to reduce or eliminate long-term pain and injury.

4 Your negative moods and attitudes will transform along with your body.

This is crucial. A game changer. You can bang away on your body all day in the gym, and if your mind and spirit aren't right, you will not reach your full potential. This program will get your mind right, because I will show you how to get your mind right. It's a path. You walk it. It's part of the program and consists of tangible exercises, just like the physical side. You work mental and spiritual muscles, just like the physical side. And just so we're clear, when I say "spiritual," I mean the internal power that drives you and inspires you, your life force, whatever you choose to call it. You want to transform your whole life? This section of the program will do that, and it'll do it in the same way: by giving you know-how, motivation, and, most important, accountability.

5 You will discover your hidden physical weaknesses—and fix them.

You may have heard of the kinetic chain, the inter-locked series of muscles and joints that runs from your feet to your fingertips. I'll get into more detail about the specifics later, but the kinetic chain in your body is the source of many of the physical problems people face today. The IMPACT program features a series of eight simple self-tests that will analyze your kinetic chain. Anyone at any fitness level can perform these. First, this battery of tests will reveal deficiencies you didn't know you had. It will show you where your body is deconditioned or out of balance. Then we let the program take over to correct those imbalances. This leads to total fitness and a high-functioning body. Remember one of my rules: You're only as strong as the weakest link in your kinetic chain.

6 Your body will shed fat, build muscle, and become a high-performance metabolic engine.

I'll introduce you to the Muscle Matrix. This is the big one. This is the whole program. A matrix is three-dimensional. And the Muscle Matrix works you in three dimensions. An example of something that doesn't work you in three dimensions: running forward in a straight line. Day after day. Mile after mile. Don't get me wrong: Running is awesome. But if done alone, this is one-dimensional training.

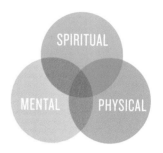

The physical, mental, and spiritual elements of your life overlap and interact. If you neglect one, you throw the entire system out of balance.

Straight ahead, very little unique challenge to the muscles. In this program, the Muscle Matrix attacks all lines of movement and gives you integrative conditioning. If you go forward, go backward. If you go left, go right. You do two legs, do one leg. Two arms, do one arm. Use rotations and diagonal actions as part of your training. This is for all athletes. All people. Look at your body as a sphere, and train the sphere at all angles. Coordination, rhythm, skipping—we begin to lose all these once we leave childhood. Starting today, you'll get them back.

You'll begin with a dynamic warmup (which will actually be a workout in itself for some people), joint integrity, strength, balance, mobility, flexibility, core conditioning, metabolic training, and more. The whole program pivots on the Muscle Matrix. The exercises are based on real, functional movements, engaging every muscle, from the big glutes to the smallest stabilizing muscles throughout your core. This is all about total-body conditioning rather than single-muscle, single-movement exercises you'll find in old-fashioned training programs. Commit to the IMPACT program and you won't blow out your back lifting a basket of laundry or yanking a suitcase out of the overhead bin of an airplane. Train like the pros, baby.

7 You will play with cutting-edge toys.

You'll see workout gear in this book that you may not have seen before. Still, most good gyms will have it. If the gym you belong to doesn't, the equipment is relatively inexpensive. You can transform a room in your house into a world-class gym for a few hundred dollars. I recommend Superbands, which are literally big rubber bands; Sport Cords, which are rubber tubing with plastic handles; and kettlebells, which come in various weights and look like cannonballs with handles. Don't be fooled—even small ones are heavy! Then there's the BOSU ball, which forces your small stabilizing muscles to fire as you use your bigger ones. (BOSU stands for "Both Sides Utilized," as in both sides of your brain, as well as "Both Sides Up," since we'll use both sides of the ball.) And you'll become a lifetime friend and fan of the TRX. The TRX is basically an adjustable nylon strap with two handles and attaching foot cradles. Simple. You hang it from a steel bar or over a door, a beam, a swing set, a tree branch, or anything else that gives you 6 feet of height (and won't snap!). We use the TRX for suspension training, which employs nothing but your own body weight. Trust me when I say that this device can single-handedly deliver one of the most intense workouts you'll ever have. The exercise combinations for the TRX can run into the hundreds. I'll give you the top moves that will have the greatest IMPACT.

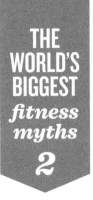

THE WORLD'S BIGGEST *fitness myths* 2

Pro athletes are the fittest people on the planet.

This story inspires everyone I tell: I wrote earlier in the book about my fitness hero, 70-year-old Donna Dickinson. Well, a couple of years ago, she and one of my pros started talking some smack while training at my facility. They ended up in a one-legged inverted Swiss-ball pushup contest. My pro athlete muscled out 9. And there goes Donna, one after the other, looking far more graceful doing hers than he did. She rattled off 15!

I tell this story because it proves that "regular folks" can do the same exercises that pros do, can train with the same intensity as the pros, and can excel like the pros, even if they don't have the same body makeup or athletic ability. That's why I train all my clients with the same IMPACT program.

8 You'll eat delicious, mouthwatering food and still lose weight.

Eating habits are the biggest saboteur of any fitness program. I keep it simple: In the IMPACT program, you're gonna eat. You'll feed your hungry muscles, have nutrients seeping into every molecule, and feel great throughout the day. You will learn the keys to proper nutrition, and I guarantee there are concepts here—such as my 90-10 rule—that you've never heard before. They are not hard to follow. Without them, you will not get the results you want. It's that simple.

9 You will bounce back faster and stronger from hard workouts.

The bottom line of any fitness program is to tear down the body. When we rest and refuel, our bodies repair themselves and come back stronger. This program optimizes that process. Obviously we talk about fuel, consuming only the premium gasoline for our high-performance engine. But you also have to take sleep seriously. Most of our body repair and regeneration takes place during sleep. When you get enough sleep, you're giving your body the proper time and resources to rebuild itself.

The program will show you other simple ways to help your body bounce back: supplements (what and when); massage therapy and bodywork; active recovery days; nontraining days. This is all the stuff that supports, reinforces, and enhances the payoff of your workouts.

10 You will eliminate every last excuse for not working out.

Man, I love eliminating excuses. Love it. And one of the whoppers is "I don't have time/equipment/ knowledge to work out." Guess what? I know what that's like. I travel a ton. I have a wife and three kids. I'm running my training facility. Going like mad all day long. How about you? Clocking millions in frequent flyer mileage? Driving the family minivan all day? Sitting in too many meetings? Stuck in client dinners that go till 10 p.m.? Well, I have a whole section devoted to quick, powerful IMPACT workouts for you. All you need is 10 or 20 minutes and your own body weight to work with. And if you want something just as fast but even more intense? Oh yeah. I have you covered there, too.

It's time to roll, baby! Game on. I can't make it any simpler for you. Let's get your mind right and get started—10 in—10 out!

"You can't choose your potential, but you can choose to fulfill it."

—THEODORE ROOSEVELT

3
GET YOUR MIND RIGHT

 "The pessimist sees difficulty in every opportunity. The optimist sees opportunity in every difficulty."

—WINSTON CHURCHILL

DO NOT SKIP THIS CHAPTER.

I know you're probably eager to skip ahead to the workouts, the cool pictures, the new exercises and toys. But the "exercises" in this chapter are essential if you want to get to the next level in your fitness and your life. They are just as critical and will deliver just as dramatic results as anything else you do in a workout. These are game-changing moves. Neglect them and you'll continue to get what you've always gotten, because you'll continue to do what you've always done. Shortcut a program? Walk away early? Fail again?

That ends today. Today we start getting your mind right.

Remember what I told you about Dub Leigh? The story didn't end there. After he finished driving his elbows into my hips during that sixth session, coughing, calling me dummy, and telling me how toxic I was, I got off the table and couldn't believe how good I felt. This was different from the other sessions. There would be no vomiting—from that day forward, Vicodin would be just a bad memory. I flexed my knees, jumped up and down with a little pogo hop. And I said, "Dub! I feel unbelievable! I don't feel any pain. I think I can play football again."

WHACK! Dub Leigh backhanded me across the face and said, "No, dodo bird! Your time is done. Your playing days are over. Get it out of your head. The lesson that you learned ended your football career. Now your work is to share what you learned with the millions of people who need to be helped. My work is being passed on to you so you can share it with others."

Let me tell you, when someone you respect smacks you across the face and rips into you like this, it cuts deep. I'd never been hit like that before, and it was exactly what I needed. My mind hadn't been right through my entire injury ordeal. I'd been just like many other self-involved men and women who ignore the warning signs and pop pills, hoping the pain will go away. After all the agony, the misery, the work to get back to health, I still always had it in the back of my mind that if I could fix my back, maybe I could play again. I'd been kidding myself—and it took a backhand across the face from an 80-year-old man for me to realize that it was time to move on to the next phase of my life. My own example is one of the best I can give to prove to you that you cannot start any kind of life transformation if your mind is not right.

That's what I say to my clients when I can tell they're not present even when they're standing in front of me. "Get your mind right." Because it's true what they say about sports. The biggest part of the game takes place between your ears. Finally, once and for all, get your mind right.

How do you get your mind right? Where do you begin?

FIRST UNDERSTAND YOURSELF. Working in the fitness field, I can say that one of the biggest mental hurdles holding people back from real success is a limiting belief system. Maybe it was the way you were raised, or the people surrounding you, or a lack of self-confidence, or even fear—there are many causes. If you nurture limiting beliefs, they'll rule your behavior and your life. I've heard it all:

"I'm not athletic enough to do an IMPACT kind of workout." (So I don't have to.)

"Your attitude determines your altitude."

— ZIG ZIGLAR

"I've never been able to lose the fat in my thighs/belly." (So I won't try.)

"Women shouldn't work with weights—I'll get all bulked up." (So I'll stick to the treadmill.)

"I have a bad back; I have to be careful what activity I do." (So I'll remain sedentary.)

"I'm afraid to change because . . ." (Nothing changes!)

These examples illustrate how people allow self-defeating thoughts to rule their activity, and in turn, their fitness, their well-being, their ultimate ability to succeed. Limiting belief systems are learned behaviors. But if you can learn it, you can also unlearn it. This chapter will help you smash through all those obstacles.

To attack your limiting belief systems, realize that you must work on strengthening your mindset first. If your mental, emotional, and spiritual side—your inner self—is out of shape, you'll never find the kind of success in life you hope to find—no matter how hard you work your body. This means you have to condition your inner self the same way you condition your outer self—with specific exercises designed to help you.

This program isn't just about how you look—though a little vanity is just fine if it helps keep you motivated in the gym. It's about how you feel, how you perform, what you can achieve. We're emotional and spiritual beings. How you look is a sweet side effect of how the IMPACT program affects your physical capabilities, your mental toughness, your ability to achieve. And what's one of the biggest problems we all face? We're emotionally overstressed and physically under-stressed. We live sedentary lives while never dragging our emotional garbage to the curb—anxiety, disappointment, anger, frustration, you name it. We steep in our own stress hormones, doing nothing to release the pain. So you have to train inwardly just as aggressively as you train outwardly.

In high school, I once played basketball against a remarkable coach at an inner-city high school in Lakewood, New Jersey. Coach John "Pott" Richardson was huge—6-foot-6, black, his head shaved shiny. He always wore a suit and had this gold pendant hanging around his neck that said "P.M.A." in big letters. "Positive mental attitude"—He instilled it in his players every single day, whether it was basketball season or not. He was relentless with his message: If you want to be the best, you must maintain a positive mental attitude at all times. That's what I'm talking about.

Positive mental attitude is just one trait of a high performer. Some others: vision, commitment, passion, discipline, mental toughness, and a burning desire to fulfill your potential. These form the foundation of high performance.

And low performers? No vision. Laziness,

IMPACT SECRETS
from the pros

KEVIN BURNETT
LINEBACKER
SAN DIEGO CHARGERS

Todd Durkin client for 2 years

WHY HE NEEDS IMPACT TRAINING: "The thing about Todd is that he knows how to get the best of you. It's in his energy, his workouts, and his intensity. Todd is someone who can tell you what you should be doing, and is willing to help you do what it takes to become better."

WHEN HE REALIZED IMPACT MADE A DIFFERENCE: "There's no one moment. It's literally every time I see Todd. The workouts with Todd are never the same. It helps prevent your body from adapting, the workouts from going stale, and it makes you a better conditioned athlete. Every time I see Todd, I know that I have to be ready for anything, and that helps build confidence that I can take on other challenges."

HIS TRAINING SECRET: "Finding a program that targets your weakness is important, but it's just as important to be able to do the type of exercise you love. It makes it easier to stay motivated and want to become better. The more interested you are in what you're doing, the harder you'll work, and the better your results will be."

apathy, a bad habit of blaming everyone else for their own problems, and a phone-book-size catalog of excuses for every occasion. These form the foundation of all limiting belief systems.

Any of them ring a bell?

Time for a little "get your mind right" training. I'm going to introduce you to a few exercises that will help you train your mind the way you'll train your body. Exercises that will help you supercharge your attitude and overcome low performance tendencies. Exercises that will help you change your entire life.

First, we start with a GCM—the Game-Changing Move. It's an absolute requirement for success, it won't take long to do—and you only have to do it once. Not daily, not weekly. One time, just before you start the 10-week IMPACT program. It'll take you about an hour. If you have to, you can even substitute it for one of your workouts. That's not ideal, but that's how important this is.

When you're finished, I'll tell you about some favorite low-effort/high-payoff additions to your life: new ideas or just new ways to get the most out of the positive things you may already be doing. None of these other activities take more than 10 minutes. Each one is like icing on a cake.

60 Minutes That Will Change Your Life

Why do so many people fail at their new fitness or nutrition plans? It's because they haven't

> ## "You be the change you wish to see in the world."
>
> — MAHATMA GANDHI

fully committed to them and added the element of accountability. It's time for you and me to talk about that.

Honoring commitment and accountability is a meat-and-potatoes trait of the high-character, high-performing individual. If you want to shift from low performance to high performance, this section will cement that transformation.

I learned the meaning of commitment and accountability when I was a student-athlete at The College of William & Mary in Virginia. At the first football practice of the year, every year, all hundred guys in the football program had to stand

---

The Motivator /// Remember what I said about things you don't like? You don't like something because you need to do it. If you continue with the short exercises in this chapter, you will get your mind right. So dig in. Commit. Teach yourself to think like a champion.

up individually and publicly declare in front of their teammates, "I commit to football for 199_," and you would say the year. Coach Laycock established a public commitment from every player, season to season. And it worked. It set the tone.

Now it's time for you to commit: 60 minutes total—three essential exercises that will commit you to the IMPACT program and hold you accountable to that commitment. Think of this as a workout. Your first inward workout.

Three Exercises That Will Get Your Mind Right

EXERCISE #1: Take a personal "now" inventory. Set a timer for 20 minutes and write down what you think and how you currently feel about your life. Be honest. Answer questions like What do I look like right now? How do I feel right now? How do I feel about my physical conditioning? What frustrates me most about my health, fitness, and nutrition habits? What can I do better? What about the quality of my life overall? How do I feel about my relationships? My career? My finances? My peer group? My spiritual life? How long since I've had fun and adventure? And, most important, What would I like to change? Write and write and write some more. If you go past 20 minutes, that's okay. Write down how you feel, and keep it honest.

Did you do it? Congratulations—you're a third of the way done. Now take what you've written and save it. It's a snapshot, a little piece of history that you will appreciate after you've finished the IMPACT program. Later, you'll reread it and see just how far you've come.

EXERCISE #2: Make your decree. This is the big one. Don't skimp on this. It's one of the cornerstones of the entire IMPACT program.

WRITE IN A JOURNAL

INVEST IN A notebook or journal and write for 10 minutes a day. Why? Writing about a feeling or a goal is far more powerful than just thinking about it, or even talking about it. Writing focuses you on the thought. Writing creates awareness and clarity. Writing builds connections. Writing reinforces. Ten minutes a day. 10 in—10 out.
JOURNAL JUMP-STARTERS: For those of you new to this activity, these tips will get you started. This is pretty powerful stuff.

- My goals for the coming week are . . .
- One new way to improve my time management habits is . . .
- Patterns I can see in my actions, feelings, or moods are . . .
- The high point of the past week was . . .
- My biggest motivator is . . .
- Where I see the most progress is . . .
- The one most difficult thing for me is . . .
- I can turn my positive progress outward to other people in my life by . . .
- My theme/focus this week will be . . .
- I'm thankful for . . .

Remember, with journaling, the sky's the limit.

Here's a secret: I run into people who have trained all their lives and have never gotten anywhere. The main reason is they don't know where they're going. They have no specific vision. You must have a vision. You must write it down. You must make it your DECREE.

What's a decree? It's a statement, typically several paragraphs long, that announces to the

> # "Nothing great was ever achieved without enthusiasm."
>
> — RALPH WALDO EMERSON

world—or at least to you—what you want to happen for your life. Decrees can be set for 10 years, 1 year, or whatever time period you would like to cover. Today, we will be doing a 10-Week Decree.

Your decree is your power source. It's the basis of your commitment and your accountability. A successful decree should move you, stir your soul, give you a positive emotional charge whenever you see it or think about it. It's not a simple goal-setting exercise. This is something you will read every morning to inspire you to get moving, to get 1 percent better every day.

Now you see why I call it your Game-Changing Move. A great decree is a game changer.

So . . . how do you write one? First, reread your personal "now" inventory—the description you just completed of how you feel today. Now, I want you to fast-forward 10 weeks and envision how

you will look and feel then. I want you to see the new you. The IMPACT you. What do you look like? What do you feel like? What is your life like?

You're creating a vision. You're making a public, or at least a personal, statement about how your life will look in 10 weeks. That's powerful.

Need some writing tips? Ten weeks from now: How many days a week are you exercising? What are you eating? How is your energy? How much do you weigh? What changes have you made to your personal life? How are your relationships going? What changes have you made in how you approach your job? What are you doing differently to live a more fulfilling life?

Here's the key: Write it down as if it has already occurred. Imagine 10 weeks from now, when you are looking back and reflecting on your journey.

I'll help get you started. Begin with this sentence and just keep writing: "I am so happy and thankful now that _____."

Remember, it's 10 weeks from today, and the changes you desire have occurred. You made it, and your vision is complete. What does your success look like? What does it feel like? Write a very clear statement—a few paragraphs in the present tense—of what you want to occur in your life.

Please don't skip this exercise. High-character people with high-performance tendencies honor their commitments. It's too easy to just say to yourself, "I'm really going to stick to this plan," and then your fire burns out after a few days or a couple of weeks, just as it does with so many other people. Quitters don't have decrees.

Your decree creates accountability. That's why you write it. Writing it reinforces it and gives it strong emotion and power. It must be on paper. You must see it. Whenever I make a decree, I write it and I share it with my wife, Melanie. That way, it's out there. I can't take it back or let it slide or forget about it. *Commit. Now.*

A Sample Decree

"I am so grateful and happy now that I've found balance in my life. I am exercising 5 days a week, I weigh 180 pounds, and I have more energy than ever. I eat five smaller, healthy meals each day, and I'm going to bed before 11:00 p.m. 7 days a week. It has been a huge step to eliminate sodas and alcohol from my diet. I'm alert and feel energetic throughout the day.

"Even better, my focus on physical conditioning has jump-started other parts of my life. My spouse and I are doing a date night every week, and we have a newfound spark that had been missing. I'm thankful for the quality time I spend each day with my kids. We got away over a long weekend in the past 10 weeks, and it was one of the most memorable trips we've ever taken as a family.

"My morning routine has been just awesome. I start off every day with a 10-minute meditation, I write for about 10 minutes, and then most days I get in a solid workout. I feel great!

"Lastly, I'm so much more relaxed at work, and I feel that my relationships there have improved. All in all, I am just happy and grateful. While life still has its challenges and adversities, I am so much stronger and better able to deal with them."

EXERCISE #3: Summarize your decree. When you're finished writing your decree, I want you to condense it down so that it fits onto an index card. Select the key words that dig deep into your emotional core and move you, inspire you, make you want to turn loose another day's worth of world-class performance in everything you do. This is your IMPACT card. Carry it with you. Use it. Read it every morning. Think of it as a ticket to a transformed life.

You've written your decree. You have a vision.

You're doing the work to get your mind right. Earlier on, I promised you some icing on this cake, and here it is. Five low-effort, high-impact opportunities that will nourish your soul, motivate your spirit, tap into your inner strength, and energize you like nothing else.

▶ 1 **LISTEN TO GREAT MUSIC.** The right music at the right time can shift a negative mindset to a positive one. Music moves your soul—and helps get your mind right. Music can help you work out harder and better. Music can fire you up for a big event. You know when you need it. Have it at the ready.

▶ 2 **READ GREAT BOOKS**. Hey, you're reading a great book right now! But seriously, read as many books as you can get your hands on. Reading engages the mind on a different level because it takes you out of your present (stress!) and into a different world full of different experiences. It pushes aside negative thoughts and feelings. It awakens ideas. And don't forget about audiobooks. You spend hundreds of hours each year in the car—why waste the time?

▶ 3 **MEDITATE.** Meditation is simple but powerful. And you don't need a huge chunk of time for it. Start with 10 minutes. You don't even have

to call it meditation. Call it quiet time, breathing time, prayer, whatever you want. A life coach I work with, Robin Sharma, calls it "the Holy Hour," because it is sacred.

Once you've established the time and place, all you really need to do is breathe. In. Out. In. Out. Let your thoughts go where they want to go. Don't direct them. Your mind will take care of itself if you step away and just observe it, so to speak. Give it time and space to reorganize and replenish itself. Ten minutes is all it takes. But take more if you want.

Do this a few days in a row and you'll start to feel so terrific you won't miss a day.

▶ 4 **WORK OUT HARD.** Yes, I know I said this chapter was all about conditioning your inner self, but your workouts are an integral part of that. If you feel stressed, anxious, angry, all balled up in the belly, hit a workout hard. Feel those endorphins surge through your body and soothe your soul. Your mind is always right after a hard workout.

▶ 5 **TRAIN YOUR BRAIN TO ATTACK LIMITING BELIEFS AND NEGATIVE THOUGHTS.** It's so easy to slip into a negative mindset, especially if it has been your way for years. But if you commit (there's that word again!) to eliminating those tendencies in yourself, you will gradually change from a low performer to a high performer. Do all of these simple exercises regularly during the day and you'll see results.

• Seek out positive people. What if your best friend is the most negative person in the world? Make an effort to meet and engage positive-minded, high-performing people. They lift you up and show you the way every time.

• Find your trigger. Whenever you think or act negatively, give yourself a signal—snap a rubber band around your wrist, put a quarter in a jar, something relevant to you alone that reminds you what you're trying to accomplish. As these moments occur, try to discover your personal negativity triggers—a certain person, world news, politics, whatever sets you off. Once you discover them, you can better handle them.

• Post inspiring quotes. Motivation comes from motivators. For me, that means powerful quotes. I love quotes. You'll see "IMPACT Quotes" throughout this book. Put them everywhere. Let them engage you and elevate your thinking.

I've said from the get-go that IMPACT is an action-oriented plan. Take action. Ready, fire, aim. The short exercises in this chapter will get you in touch with and keep you connected to your emotional and spiritual self, your inner strength. It's all about you and the stuff that's buried inside that maybe you don't fully understand right now. But you will, I promise you. Do the work. Get your mind right!

"Just as your car runs smoothly and requires less energy to run faster and farther when the wheels are in alignment, you perform better when your thoughts, feelings, emotions, goals, and values are in balance."

—BRIAN TRACY

4
SECRETS TO A
PAIN-FREE BODY

 "It's not whether you get knocked down, it's whether you get up."
—VINCE LOMBARDI

Why do our bodies hurt so much?

That's not just a good question; it's an important one. Sometimes we have pain and we have no idea what we did to cause it. And pain holds us back from so much. Maybe you want to lose weight, but your knees hurt. Or you want to change your body shape, but your back and neck hurt. Or maybe you already have a good level of strength and fitness but experience nagging injuries and pain that prevent you from getting to the next level. I know what that feels like.

The secrets in this chapter will help you feel better.

Secrets? I call them secrets because not many people know about them or use them to help themselves break the pain cycle. If you have pain, what do you usually do? Rest. Medicate. This doesn't typically solve the root of the problem. You haven't found the answer because you're looking in all the wrong places. I introduced you to fascia and the kinetic chain in Chapter 2. Knowledge about the fascial system and its important connection to the kinetic chain will give you the power to end the pain cycle and create real change in your life.

The basics are worth repeating: Fascia is a tough, cobweb-like sheath that envelops our muscles, nerves and bones. There's nothing mystical or mysterious about it. It's an actual, physical substance that you would see if you could look beneath your skin. Fascia supports your organs and joints from head to toe and acts as a shock absorber.

In its natural state, fascia is elastic, pliable, and relaxed. However, fascia often becomes constricted due to trauma, accident, repetitive motion syndrome, neuromuscular weakness, or poor posture. Fascia shrinks when inflamed and is slow to heal because of poor blood supply. When fascia tightens, it creates great pressure on the tissue it surrounds, inhibits motion and flexibility, and becomes a significant source of tension in the body. Fascia also has a generous supply of nerves.

This means if you are hurting or your body is a wreck, you will feel pain.

In the world of performance enhancement and pain management, fascia has been thought of as "the bag that holds the gold coins [muscle]." Who would have thought the bag might be just as precious as the gold?

In this chapter, you'll learn two primary ways to feel better: how to treat your fascia, and how to address the things in your daily life that are causing your pain. That includes challenging the way you think about movement and exercise. This chapter will introduce you to the kinetic chain—how your body really works—and show you how this system functions hand-in-hand with fascia. The 10-minute foam roller ritual in these pages—good for preworkout or stand-alone use—will prevent further injuries and can help heal your chronic pain.

The Kinetic Chain

Did you know that your nagging knee pain could be caused by tight muscles in your hips? Or that your neck pain and headaches could come from badly conditioned thoracic muscles?

You might wonder, "How can tight muscles in one part of my body make an unrelated part hurt?" The answer: Your entire body is related and compensates for imbalance, pain, or injury in order to protect itself. Every part is completely linked and dependent on every other part through a system called the kinetic chain. We can't understand sources of pain until we understand

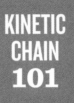

KINETIC CHAIN 101

Optimal performance of the kinetic chain comes from two interrelated principles that must cooperate for the system to function properly.

STABILITY: The muscle, tendon, and ligament action needed to hold a joint in position.

MOBILITY: Joint movement, encompassing both the ability of the joint to move through its largest, safest range of motion and the ability of the nearby muscles to cause that motion.

the important working relationship between fascia and the kinetic chain.

What is the kinetic chain? Well, kinetic means movement (you probably learned about kinetic energy, the energy produced by movement, in sixth-grade science class). Your kinetic chain is the system that promotes movement—from feet to fingertips—and the muscles, fascia, and other connective tissues that tie it all together. Some of it is designed for mobility, some for stability. This collection of parts functions as one, each part depending on the others for optimal performance. If one area is weak, another part must compensate, and the system suffers. If one part is not mobile and is supposed to be, another part compensates, and the next link will suffer. That's why you're only as strong as the weakest link in your kinetic chain.

Please take a look at the sidebar on how the kinetic chain functions. Do you notice a pattern? The components of the kinetic chain alternate between stability and mobility. That's how it works so well: One part supports the movement of another—the same way 11 members of the best offense in the NFL work as one cohesive unit for optimum performance.

If one component of the kinetic chain is broken or deficient, your body will compensate, and you will end up in pain. If your tight hips can't move, your spine will. If your foot is not stable, it can affect your knees, hips, back . . . your entire body.

And while every joint plays a critical role in the health of your body, I want you to focus an extra moment on your hips. If your hips are tight and can't function correctly, you're on the road to pain and injury. Talk with any bodywork professional whose clients include elite athletes—football, baseball, golf, tennis, you name it. They'll all say it doesn't matter what sport or position, or even what the presenting symptom is. The hips are always tight!

The Six Most Common Causes of Chronic Daily Pain

These are the everyday things you do that cause you pain—and you may not even know you're doing them. Fascia is intimately involved with each one. Simply knowing these things can be a weapon against them, but for good measure I'll also give you smart tips for addressing the most common things that wreck our bodies. What are they?

- **Elevated stress**
- **Too much sitting**
- **HRD** (Don't know what that is? Keep reading.)
- **Poorly designed exercise programs**
- **Too little stretching**
- **Poor recovery and regeneration**

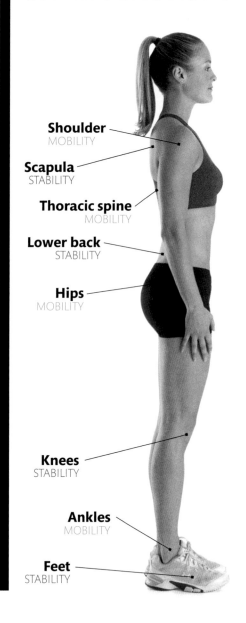

HOW THE KINETIC CHAIN FUNCTIONS:

Shoulder
MOBILITY

Scapula
STABILITY

Thoracic spine
MOBILITY

Lower back
STABILITY

Hips
MOBILITY

Knees
STABILITY

Ankles
MOBILITY

Feet
STABILITY

#1 ELEVATED STRESS There are two kinds of stress: eustress (positive) and distress (negative). Yes, there actually is "good" stress, and we need it in our lives to perform optimally, because stress is married to performance. Think about the stress you feel as you square up with the golf ball on the 18th tee on a Sunday afternoon. You're down a stroke. Competing against your friends. You think, "Yeah baby, let's sink this thing!" This is positive stress. With it, you rise to a challenge.

Distress, on the other hand, is essentially negative. Excessive dis-stress will lead to dis-ease. Your typical day is filled with stressors: a commute, work responsibilities, chores at home, meal preparation, family and friends—in other words . . . life. Some demands always create negative stress (tight deadlines at work, a sick child, an argument with a spouse or loved one, doing your taxes, etc.). But sometimes even good demands become too many and eustress becomes distress.

When you live in excessive distress, you feel anxiety, anger, irritability, and frustration. Emotions activate your body's fight-or-flight system, releasing stress hormones such as adrenaline and cortisol. This wreaks havoc on your body. Your blood pressure spikes. Your breathing becomes shallow. And bingo: Your muscles from your neck down through your back tense up. Tightness. Discomfort. Headaches. Pain.

#2 TOO MUCH SITTING Not many people are able to make a living on their feet these days. So you sit—in front of computers, in meetings, at lunch, on the couch at night. You spend hours in one position. Your hips, hamstrings, and quads have no way to move. Your glutes take the brunt of your weight. Your chest muscles tighten and pull your shoulders forward. Your neck, shoulders, and back tense up, and you slump and hunch forward. You can't stay properly aligned, because sitting for hours promotes lousy posture. Poor posture

THE WORLD'S BIGGEST *fitness myths* 3

I'll never be flexible—my muscles have been tight all my life.

THE TRUTH: You make yourself inflexible by never training for it. This can happen from not exercising, of course, but also from exercising improperly and causing muscle imbalances (working your chest more than your back, for example).

Sometimes inflexibility or tightness isn't the problem. Maybe it's your fascia, or you might have unstable muscles—in your core, for example —that restrict your full range of motion and put a "brake" on certain movements. If you properly condition your core, you'll move easier and have greater range of motion—and appear to be more flexible. Train your weaknesses and you will improve.

alters your body's fascia and limits its elasticity. That's a recipe for perpetual pain.

#3 HRD What is that? HRD stands for hip rotational deficit, and it may be killing your structural system. Our hips play a critical role in how our bodies feel and function. And when I am talking hips, I'm talking about the hip external rotator muscles (glutes and piriformis), the hip internal rotator muscles (primarily the psoas and groin muscles), and the hip flexor muscles (primarily the psoas muscles).

The entire hip complex plays a major role in how the body functions. The intricate relationship between the hip flexors and hip rotators also dictates how the pelvis functions. And there are dozens of small muscles around the pelvis that help us flex and rotate the trunk, as well as stabilize the back. All these muscles are connected by fascia.

Renowned movement specialist Moshe Feldenkrais once said, "You go as your pelvis goes." When your pelvis is off level, out of balance, rotated, tilted forward or back, or not sitting perfectly, your body is compromised. And when this happens, it negatively impacts the length and tension of the muscles and fascia, which will in turn cause the body to move inefficiently. Because of the compensatory actions of the kinetic chain, before you know it, you have several joints hurting, and you end up in pain.

Therefore, mobility and flexibility of the muscles surrounding the pelvis and hips are critical to keeping the body pain free, performing well, and feeling great.

The IMPACT program targets all these areas to help protect your hips and ensure balance and flexibility throughout your entire body.

#4 POORLY DESIGNED EXERCISE PROGRAMS

I am convinced the football injury that ended my career was simply "the straw that broke the camel's back." Yes, two linebackers speared me in the back with their helmets. But, at the same time, the strength and conditioning program I was doing back then didn't take into account hip mobility, lower-back stability, and midthoracic mobility. At all. I lacked proper rotational training, core strength, and flexibility. And ultimately I was more susceptible to injury.

Yes, I know you might be working out. But have you ever thought that you might be doing some movements in your program that are exacerbating the conditions that cause your pain? Do you work your back side at least as often as your front side? I recommend a minimum of a 1:1 back-to-front ratio. That means for every "push" exercise you do, you ideally do at least one "pull" exercise. In the

HOW DO YOU KNOW IF YOU HAVE HRD?

TAKE THESE TESTS FROM
KAHL GOLDFARB, PT, DPT, OMT, CSCS

TEST YOUR INTERNAL HIP ROTATION.

LIE ON YOUR right side in the fetal position and place a towel between your knees. Keeping your knees in contact with the towel, lift your left foot off your right foot as far as possible. Then lie on your left side and repeat with your right foot, and compare. The distance between feet each time should be equal. If not, you may have hip internal rotational deficit, or HIRD.

TEST YOUR EXTERNAL HIP ROTATION WITH THE PIGEON POSE.

GET ON ALL FOURS, straighten your right leg, and slide it back, behind, and across your left leg. Move your left foot forward to further stretch your hips. Place your hands on the floor in front of your left leg and slowly bring your torso down into a forward bend with your chest as close as possible to your left knee. Be sure to keep your hips squared with the floor. Let the weight of your body rest on your left leg, and breathe. You should feel the stretch in your left glute.

Switch sides and compare your hips. If one side feels significantly different or you experience pain in your hip joint, you may have hip external rotational deficit, or HERD. This means you must emphasize a stretching and mobility program for your glutes and piriformis. If you have pain inside the joint, you should seek medical advice.

In either test, if one hip is significantly tighter than the other, you need to emphasize a hip mobility and flexibility program.

athlete training world, we say the "mirror" muscles, such as the biceps, chest, and abs, make you "all show and no go." Sure, you look good, but you'll never perform to your full potential. Improve your fitness and sports performance—get some "steak with your sizzle"—by working the back side of your body as much as your front side.

Most traditional workout programs are linear based. They train in one plane of action. Running, cycling, and rowing are primarily performed in a straight line. And most machines isolate muscles in only one fixed plane of motion. Yet your body typically moves in multiple planes and multiple dimensions. Shouldn't your program mimic real life?

#5 **TOO LITTLE STRETCHING** There is no way to sugarcoat it. The average person, even the average active person, has serious flexibility issues, especially in the hips, hamstrings, and chest. The older you get, the worse it becomes. Think about it. When time is tight, what part of your workout do you skip? Bingo. Stretching. You know the drill by now. Failure to stretch properly leads to muscle tightness, discomfort, pain, injury. There's that wreck of a body again.

#6 **POOR RECOVERY AND REGENERATION**
If you change the way you exercise, that's a good start. It's part of the equation. But you can't fix your body with workouts alone. You need to rest and recover. Allow your body to reenergize. Nutrition, sleep, and flexibility all play a role in this process. (You'll learn more about it in Chapter 9.) The main point is this: Your recovery needs to be an active process. You have to work hard in order to help your body cope with all the daily stresses—including those you purposely create (like exercise) and those you don't (injury and daily frustrations). Repetitive motion syndrome is a chief cause of constricted fascia. I'll say it again: Rest. Recover. Reenergize.

WHY WE HURT AND *how to prevent it*

By Kahl Goldfarb, PT, DPT, OMT, CSCS

The body utilizes all joints during normal motion. A restriction in one joint, such as the hip, can result in increased stress placed on adjacent body parts or joints. The cumulative result over time can be degenerative disk disease, a herniated disk, sciatica, degenerative joint disease (which can lead to a hip or knee replacement), knee cartilage tears, IT band syndrome, runner's knee, or even plantar fasciitis. Addressing the muscular issue, fascial restriction, or joint tightness in the hip can prevent many of these problems from developing.

For Every Problem, There Is a Solution

Here's the deal. Your body may be a wreck. And your daily habits are largely to blame. The good news is there are solutions. But they require change. Change will come with knowledge and effort. In other words, understand your body and do the work. The human body is amazing. Graceful in movement. Incredibly strong. Unbelievably resilient. Amazing to watch. Beautiful. Healthy fascia is an essential ingredient. Without healthy fascia, we aren't graceful because we're tight. We aren't resilient because we're prone to injury. We aren't amazing because we are in pain.

Keep reading. You're gonna feel better.

You need to pay close attention to this section on solutions. Practice all of them—they are the keys to banishing pain from your life.

WHEN YOU SPEND LONG HOURS AT A DESK, GET UP OCCASIONALLY AND STRETCH. Get out of your chair at least once every 2 hours and walk around or stretch for 10 minutes. Do some lunges. Walk to the bathroom. Move your body.

And while you are sitting? Be aware of your posture. Prevent slumping by keeping your shoulders back and your chest open—this allows full, deep breaths. Proper sitting posture feels as if your shoulder blades are bearing the weight of your shoulders.

One other great sitting tip: Sit on a Swiss ball at the computer or at work to keep your core activated! This will help you be conscious of your posture and help you survive long stretches in front of the computer.

FOLLOW THE IMPACT PROGRAM TO THE LETTER. Exercise with movements that are forward and backward, left and right, up and down, diagonal, and rotational. Emphasize mobility, stability, flexibility, and core strength. All of this helps bring the kinetic chain back into balance. Now watch how your body improves.

STRETCH. Remember, if you don't like it, you need it. One of the reasons stretching feels so unrewarding is because you see no visible result—muscles don't get bigger, and you don't get any thinner. But trust me, if you emphasize flexibility and improve stability and mobility in the correct joints, you are going to feel so much better and improve the way you perform in all areas of your life. It all starts with the preworkout preparation that you'll complete at the beginning of every workout. Now, let me introduce you to your new best friend: the foam roller.

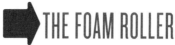

THE FOAM ROLLER

A foam roller is the best 25 bucks you'll ever spend. The 5 to 10 minutes you take for the following foam roller exercises will pay fantastic dividends. Your body will be able to move again more fluidly and freely. This quick routine is great for preworkout preparation and tune-ups between workouts.

Foam rolling is an excellent way to treat your fascia and improve its quality on a daily basis. As I told you earlier, healthy fascia is a critical element in releasing your potential. Imbalances in your fascial system need to be addressed directly, and with daily, consistent effort, foam rolling will restore your fascia to its pliable and relaxed form.

Know that rolling a tight muscle may cause discomfort. This usually means the area needs the attention. Work at it slowly. Roll back and forth in small movements to create a release. Each time you use your foam roller makes the next time a little easier. And don't forget to breathe!

FOAM ROLL SIDE-LYING SIDE OPENER

Lie on your right side on a foam roller, both legs bent 90 degrees. The foam roller should be perpendicular to your body, and just about in line with your shoulder blade. Extend your right arm overhead, roll up toward your armpit, then back to the starting position. Roll back and forth, then repeat on the other side.

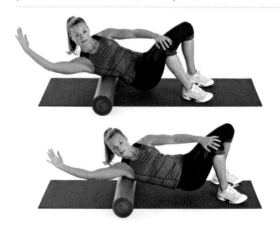

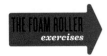
FOAM ROLL GLUTES

▶ Sit on a foam roller, with it positioned on your right glute. Cross your right leg over the front of your left thigh. Put your hands on the floor for support. Roll your body forward and backward in small movements from your lower glute to your upper glute. Repeat with the roller under your left glute.

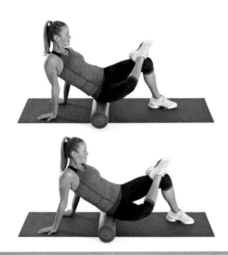

FOAM ROLL ILIOTIBIAL-BAND (IT-BAND)

▶ Lie on your right side and place your right hip on a foam roller. Put your hands on the floor for support. Cross your left leg over your right, and place your left foot flat on the floor. Roll your body forward and backward in small movements until the roller reaches just above your knee. Repeat on other side.

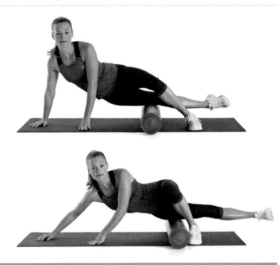

FOAM ROLL CALVES

▶ Sit on the floor with your legs stretched in front of you. Place a foam roller under your right calf. Cross your left leg over your right ankle. With your hands flat on the floor for support, raise your body off the floor while keeping your back naturally arched. Roll your body forward until the roller has crossed your entire calf. Roll back and forth. Repeat with the roller under your left calf.

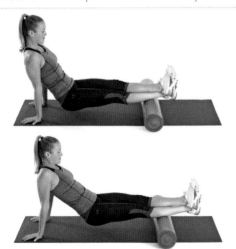

FOAM ROLL QUADS

▶ Lie facedown on the floor with a foam roller positioned just above your knees. Slowly roll your body over the roller until it reaches the tops of your thighs. Roll back and forth.

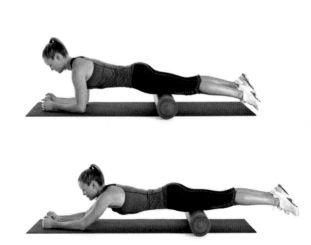

FOAM ROLL GROIN

➡ Lie facedown on the floor. Place a foam roller parallel to your body. Put your hands on the floor for support. Position your left thigh nearly perpendicular to your body, with the inner portion of your thigh just above the level of your knee, resting on top of the roller. Roll your body toward the left until the roller reaches your pelvis. Then roll back and forth. Repeat with the roller on your left thigh.

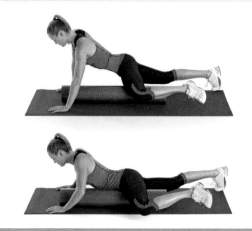

FOAM ROLL THORACIC MOBILITY

➡ Lie faceup with a foam roller under your upper back, at the tops of your shoulder blades. Cross your arms over your chest or clasp behind your head with elbows back. Your knees should be bent, with your feet flat on the floor. Raise your hips so they're slightly elevated off the floor. Roll back and forth over your shoulder blades and your mid and upper back.

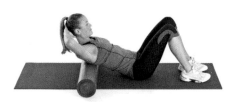

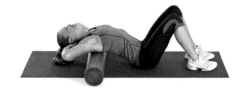

FOAM ROLL RESTORATIVE SPINE

➡ Lie faceup with a foam roller under your back, resting vertically along your spine. With your knees bent and your feet flat on the floor, reach your arms out to the sides and open up your chest. You should feel a stretch throughout the front and back of your upper body.

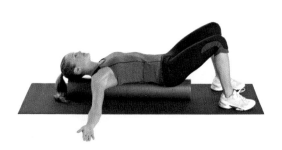

TENNIS BALL ROLLS

➡ Stand without shoes on. Roll a tennis ball from the heel of your foot to the ball of your foot. Move slowly.

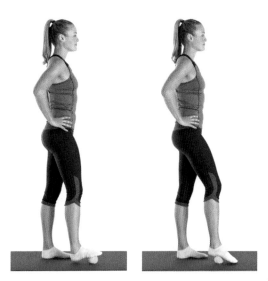

5
ENTER
THE MATRIX

"What this power is I cannot say. All I know is that it exists and it becomes available only when a man is in that state of mind in which he knows exactly what he wants and is fully determined not to quit until he finds it."

—ALEXANDER GRAHAM BELL

Few things in life can match the euphoria

you feel after a great workout. Your muscles are tired, you've worked up a serious sweat, and your mind is relaxed. And for that moment, you are free of stress and worry, and everything feels amazing! The Muscle Matrix—this chapter—is the ignition key to the IMPACT program: your introduction to the blueprint of the IMPACT workouts, how to maximize the benefit of every single exercise, and what equipment you need to make it all happen. You'll walk out of this chapter knowing everything you need to know about how to achieve world-class workouts.

The Muscle Matrix is based on more than 15 years of experience, scientific research, and daily discoveries "in the trenches" at my performance facility, Fitness Quest 10. It all adds up to a success-driven program that's been used by thousands of people to reach their goals—including some of the finest athletes in the world. I've formulated each workout to give you the best of what I know. Now it's time to tap into that knowledge for yourself.

The Muscle Matrix
Part One
||||||||||||||||||||||||||||||||||||||||||||||||||||||||||||||||||||||

THE ANATOMY OF THE MATRIX

The Muscle Matrix is a simplified system that utilizes advanced training principles to deliver maximum results. It combines training in different planes of motion (up and down, forward and back, side-to-side, diagonally, and with rotation), performing some exercises with only one arm or leg, and challenging your entire body in a diverse training environment. Unlike most traditional programs, it goes beyond just working on machines and exercising at one speed. It will challenge you to be your very best!

Just as you wouldn't go straight from learning simple addition and subtraction to performing advanced calculus, the Muscle Matrix follows an integrative, systematic approach that increases in difficulty as your body adjusts and improves. The Matrix consists of seven different components, or phases: dynamic warmup, joint integrity, core conditioning, strength and conditioning, power and plyometrics, movement training, and flexibility. You go through each phase in every workout, as they all serve a purpose in helping you reach your potential.

WHAT IS THE MUSCLE MATRIX?

The Muscle Matrix uses three dimensions to target your strengths and weaknesses. Rather than focus on just one aspect of fitness, the Muscle Matrix delivers results, guarantees a challenge, and provides diversity and fun through:

1 A seven-phase approach to training

2 Specialized methodologies and techniques that maximize the effectiveness of each exercise and workout

3 Game-changing equipment to build a high-performance body

1 Dynamic Warmup

A great workout starts with a great warmup. My friends, I have news for you: A warmup should not be easy. It will start "easy" but should progress to the point that when you're finished, you're ready to go full steam ahead into your workout. The warmup you'll do in this workout is based on movement and will challenge your rhythm, your coordination, and even your conditioning. It'll make you sweat. Once you're accustomed to the

---

The 7 Phases of the Muscle Matrix /// 1. Dynamic Warmup 2. Joint Integrity 3. Core Conditioning
4. Strength and Conditioning 5. Power and Plyometrics 6. Movement Training 7. Flexibility

FIRST LOOK ▸ THE DYNAMIC WARMUP

Learn these dynamic warmup moves and become familiar with them. You'll be performing them before every workout. It might look like a lot, but the process should eventually take you no longer than 7 to 10 minutes. Everything should happen under control, with good form, and with minimal rest between exercises.

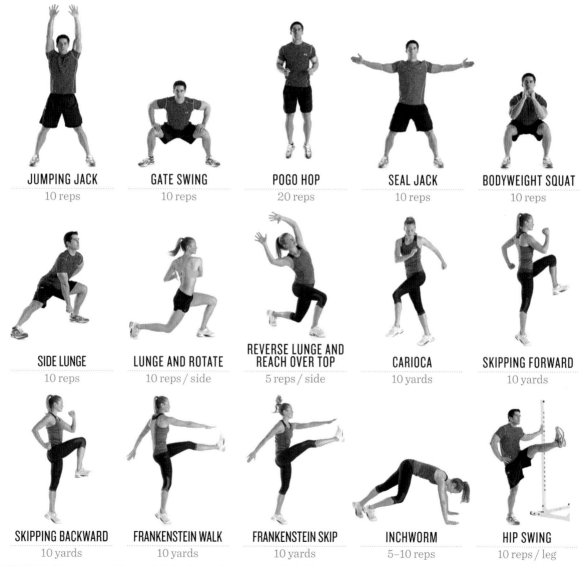

JUMPING JACK	**GATE SWING**	**POGO HOP**	**SEAL JACK**	**BODYWEIGHT SQUAT**
10 reps	10 reps	20 reps	10 reps	10 reps
SIDE LUNGE	**LUNGE AND ROTATE**	**REVERSE LUNGE AND REACH OVER TOP**	**CARIOCA**	**SKIPPING FORWARD**
10 reps	10 reps / side	5 reps / side	10 yards	10 yards
SKIPPING BACKWARD	**FRANKENSTEIN WALK**	**FRANKENSTEIN SKIP**	**INCHWORM**	**HIP SWING**
10 yards	10 yards	10 yards	5–10 reps	10 reps / leg

NOTE: This is a just a sneak peak at the more detailed workouts and instructions in the back of the book.

FIRST LOOK JOINT INTEGRITY

You'll focus on a different aspect of joint integrity in each workout. For instance, Monday might work on your hips, Wednesday on your shoulders, and Friday on your core and balance. You'll see the complete workout details in the back of the book. But your joint integrity work will look like this:

MONDAY Hips

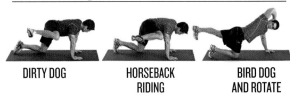

DIRTY DOG | HORSEBACK RIDING | BIRD DOG AND ROTATE

WEDNESDAY Shoulders

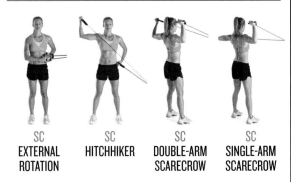

SC EXTERNAL ROTATION | SC HITCHHIKER | SC DOUBLE-ARM SCARECROW | SC SINGLE-ARM SCARECROW

FRIDAY Balance

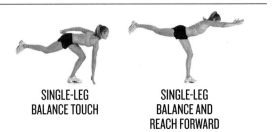

SINGLE-LEG BALANCE TOUCH | SINGLE-LEG BALANCE AND REACH FORWARD

dynamic warmup, you should be able to complete it in 7 to 10 minutes. However, starting out, many exercise rookies might feel done after the dynamic warmup. So if your idea of preparing for your workout is performing a few light sets of an exercise or walking on a treadmill for 5 minutes, you're in for a surprise.

Before you start the heart of the program, you should be sweating. A great warmup fires up your entire neuromuscular system, increases the temperature of your muscles, and lengthens your fascia. A "warm" muscle and lengthened fascia can generate more energy and force, and react more efficiently to any demand you place on them. That's why the dynamic warmup prepares your body for any movement you will perform. Your heart rate will increase, your muscles will feel loose, and your mind and body will be fully prepared for the workout. Additionally, the dynamic warmup will keep you safe and help prevent injury during your workout.
▶ **BONUS TIP:** Before each dynamic warmup, remember to improve the quality of your fascia with 5 to 10 minutes of foam rolling. Use the exercises shown in Chapter 4.

2 Joint Integrity

"If you want a monument, you must first build a strong foundation." —Tom House
The foundation of your body is your joints and ligaments; they keep you healthy and prevent injury. This includes the structures in your shoulders, core, hips, legs, and feet. Because you are only as strong as your weakest link and as efficient as your worst movement, the joint integrity portion of your workout will challenge the small, often-neglected muscles of your body. This is accomplished through a series of movements using body-weight exercises, balance work, and Sport Cords.

> *"To accomplish great things we must not only act, but also dream; not only plan, but also believe."*
>
> — ANATOLE FRANCE

---

3 Core Conditioning

Most people think of the core as their abs, but the core is the entire region from your hips up to your diaphragm and includes your lower back and obliques (you might know this area as your love handles). Your core helps stabilize your spine and plays a major role in your posture. Additionally, your core is often referred to as your power zone—with your hips, lower back, abs, and trunk generating the force when you twist, throw, or perform any action that engages your core. Your core also plays an important role in the transition of strength and power from your lower body to your upper body.

This also means a few crunches or leg raises at the end of your workout won't do the job. Your core cannot be an afterthought. It's like any other muscle in your body: It needs to be trained at multiple angles, with varying resistances, and at

THE WORLD'S BIGGEST *fitness myths* 4

Weight training bulks you up.

Women seem especially afraid of this, as if regular weight lifting will make them look like NFL linebackers. To debunk this myth, look at the female fitness model in this book. The woman in the pictures is named Anna—she works as a trainer at my facility in San Diego. And not only does she work out with weights regularly (if not religiously), she knows all the moves to the extent that she can model them with perfect technique. Now . . . does she look bulky?

The fact is, ladies, if you want to change the way your body looks and performs, you need weight training. If you want to prevent degenerative conditions like osteoporosis as you get older, you need weight training.

"Bulk" is bunk. Two things make you bulky: your diet and your training method. A specific type of training exists called sarcoplasmic hypertrophy that aims to build huge, bodybuilding-style muscles. People who train this way also need to eat massive amounts of food to fuel that muscle growth.

You won't be doing that here. Whether you're male or female, the IMPACT program will make your body look more like the respective models in the back of this book, not like a bodybuilder or an offensive lineman.

different speeds. Your abs are designed to resist movement, not create it, which is why many of the exercises in the IMPACT workout will force you to stabilize your core against outside resistance, or to use your small muscles when your body is off balance.

Although you will initially use your own body weight to work your core, you'll soon challenge your core with multiple tools, including the BOSU, TRX, and Superbands. By prioritizing your entire core early in your workout routine, you'll prioritize another common weak link in your training. This, in turn, helps your performance and allows you to swing a golf club better, improve your tennis swing, and even reveal your six-pack.

4 Strength and Conditioning

The heart of the IMPACT program builds world-class strength to maximize your potential. Ladies and gentlemen, you need resistance training to get results in any program. It doesn't matter if you're a man or a woman. Strength training improves your body from head to toe and will reinvigorate your life with energy. Sure, in IMPACT you'll do some traditional strength-training exercises using barbells and dumbbells. But the fun really starts when you incorporate kettlebells, the TRX, Superbands, the BOSU, and other new pieces of equipment. The result: You'll develop your body like never before.

Important /// The joint integrity component of the IMPACT program helps prepare your body for the increased intensity of plyometrics. Don't neglect the joint integrity section of your workouts as you progress in the program. Each movement will help keep you safe, pain free, and feeling great.

5 Power and Plyometrics

Beginning in week 4, you'll start to incorporate a technique known as plyometric training, which targets your fast-twitch muscle fibers. In the most basic sense, your body is composed of two types of muscle fibers: fast- and slow-twitch. As we age, our fast-twitch muscle fibers begin to diminish if we don't use them. This is important because we need them when an exercise or movement requires explosive power (think jumping or sprinting) or quick reaction (like playing tennis or basketball). By incorporating plyometrics in the IMPACT program, you'll trigger more fast-twitch muscle development, which will help you build more lean muscle tissue, increase your metabolism, and change your body composition.

Most plyometric exercises involve jumping or hopping because these motions force you to load your muscles (such as when you crouch down in a squat) and then quickly produce a force (explode upward). There are several variations for your lower and upper body, all of which help convert your strength into power. It's a basic equation:

Strength + speed = power.

Plyometrics can help you move more effortlessly, fluidly, and powerfully and are a big part of delivering the results you want.

6 Movement Training

I love running. I can't run like I once did, but I still enjoy the feeling of getting outside, moving my body, and pumping my arms and legs. It's a process that ignites a flow of endorphins—chemicals your brain releases during exercise—that makes your hard work feel good. This is commonly referred to as the runner's high.

IMPACT SECRETS *from the pros*

MALCOLM FLOYD
WIDE RECEIVER
SAN DIEGO CHARGERS

Todd Durkin client for 2 years

WHY HE NEEDS IMPACT TRAINING: "I came in with a lot of natural talent. Todd's honed it. And in a lot of ways, he's improved weaknesses I never knew I had. For example, he's helped me improve my posture—which doesn't sound like a big deal, but that alone helped me come out of my stance on a play more explosively. Working with Todd has made me a lot more explosive."

WHEN HE REALIZED IMPACT MADE A DIFFERENCE:
"When I touched the top of a light fixture in Todd's gym [which is about 11 feet off the floor]. He had us doing vertical jump exercises with Superbands, which gave a lot of resistance. When we finished, I jumped without the Superband, and I felt like I was flying. I touched that light and I was like, 'Oh, man!' Todd has you work muscles you never worked before."

HIS TRAINING SECRET:
"I never ignore parts of my training, even if I don't like them. I do the entire program. Why? Last season was the first season I didn't have to spend a lot of time in the trainer's room. I was healthy throughout the year. And that was my first year with Todd. I don't think that's a coincidence. That's dynamic warmup and joint integrity right there."

Running isn't the only way to release those feel-good chemicals. Anything that puts your body in motion, whether it's jogging, walking, hiking, biking, or swimming, can have you feeling much better. And that's what I want you doing in this program. Choose an activity that feels great to you, that you enjoy, and that doesn't punish your joints. While I love running, I also recommend diversifying the type of movement you perform, so you're not always doing the same thing, which can lead to overuse injuries and muscle imbalances.

The Matrix is filled with movement activities. You'll see them referenced in several ways: conditioning, grand finales, and high-intensity intervals. Even on your off days, I want you doing some sort of activity, at least one or two times a week. Just make sure you're moving and having fun. Some might call this type of exercise cardio, but that typically refers to training at one monotonous speed. To use an old-school term, we will use Fartlek training, an interval style of conditioning that means "speed play." Some days you'll move fast, some you'll move more slowly, and others it'll be a combination of the two. You might run at a steady state for 30 minutes, or take 10 minutes to sprint. The point is this: Get up and move. It's part of what makes us human and is one of the best ways to maximize your calorie burn and your results!

THE WORLD'S BIGGEST *fitness myths* 6

Cardio and resistance training are separate activities.

The thinking that you need separate cardio and resistance training days is outdated—not to mention an incredibly inefficient way to exercise. I've designed IMPACT workouts to be time efficient, comprehensive, and intense, which means you'll work your entire body hard and fast. If you train with proper intensity, trust me, IMPACT will be all the cardio you'll need (though I certainly encourage you to get out and do your favorite cardio activities in addition to IMPACT—if you love it, do it!).

That's why I talk about tempo in this chapter. An IMPACT workout is a high-tempo, high-intensity experience that will give you all the benefits of a "pure" cardio workout while also blasting every muscle in your body. Efficient, comprehensive, intense.

"I couldn't wait for success, so I went ahead without it."

— JONATHAN WINTERS

7 Flexibility

I often ask my clients what would improve the quality of their training on an ongoing basis. The most common answer: flexibility. The IMPACT program is not just about getting into great shape. It's also about becoming more flexible. To be world class with your flexibility, you need to stretch every day. This doesn't always have to be the band stretches I recommend you perform at the end of each workout, which you can find starting on page 57. It can be activities such as yoga or Pilates. Remember, when you stretch, foam roll, or work on the quality of your soft tissue, you remove adhesions that build up in your muscle fibers. These little knots not only hinder your performance, but also prevent you from feeling great. Once you start flexibility work, you'll feel looser, improve circulation, breathe better, and protect your body from injury, and ultimately your performance will improve.

The Muscle Matrix
Part Two
||||||||||||||||||||||||||||||||||||||||||||||||||||||||||||||||||

PRINCIPLES FOR MAXIMIZING EVERY EXERCISE

The seven phases of the Muscle Matrix provide the structure for each workout you'll perform. But what you'll do within the structure of the Matrix will take you beyond your average routine and into the rare territory where athletes train. The "and then some" of the Matrix occurs when you add these five training principles that allow you to supercharge your body for peak performance.

Be prepared: These principles will challenge your body like never before.

PRINCIPLE #1 **TEMPO, TEMPO, TEMPO**

One of the most challenging aspects of the IMPACT program will be the pace at which you move between exercises, and the rest periods between sets. This program is all about efficiency. I don't want you spending 2 hours in the gym, which means there's not much time to stand around and discuss your social plans for the evening. You should be focused and immersed in the activity. As a matter of fact, your tempo will allow you to complete each workout within 45 to 60 minutes. That's an excuse buster right there, baby, because the last time I checked, you were busy and didn't have all day to work out, right?

You'll do more in less time by minimizing rest and using a technique known as supersetting, which trains opposing muscle groups (such as your biceps and triceps) back-to-back, or combines a lower-body and an upper-body exercise. While one muscle group is working, the other relaxes. By going back and forth, you improve your conditioning, speed up your tempo, and still work your body just as hard but in a fraction of the time. This allows you to get in and out of the gym fast.

PRINCIPLE #2 **GIANT SETS**

When you combine three or more exercises into a "station" that you complete in a continuous fashion, it's called a giant set. The station is the group of exercises. When you complete all the reps of each exercise in the station, you've finished one round of the giant set. Sometimes a station will include as many as six exercises. And if you have to perform 2 sets, that means you'll cycle through all six exercises, rest, and then repeat the entire process.

This is an extremely time-efficient and effective way to combine multiple movements and rev up your metabolism like nothing you've ever done before, while still challenging every muscle fiber

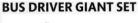

Complete 1 set of each of the three exercises as a sequence for 1 station, resting 30 seconds after each. Once you complete all three exercises (a giant set), rest for 1 to 2 minutes and then complete the station again.

BUS DRIVER GIANT SET

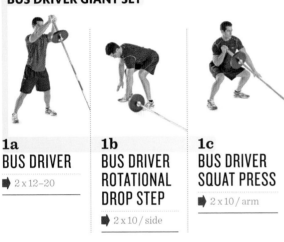

1a
BUS DRIVER
➡ 2 x 12–20

1b
BUS DRIVER ROTATIONAL DROP STEP
➡ 2 x 10 / side

1c
BUS DRIVER SQUAT PRESS
➡ 2 x 10 / arm

in your body. Try to rest a maximum of 30 to 60 seconds between exercises within the giant set, and 1 to 2 minutes after you finish each station.

PRINCIPLE #3 COMPLEX TRAINING

Complex training will help you become more explosive in your movements by combining a strength-based exercise with a plyometric exercise with little rest between the two movements. Complexes are great for developing both strength and speed, which results in power. They also challenge your muscles by taking a relatively simple move, such as a body-weight exercise, and

having you perform it when fatigued. Doing an incline dumbbell bench press immediately followed by a plyometric pushup is an example of a complex pairing. Another example would be walking lunges immediately followed by squat jumps. Complexes really put you to the test. You'll begin to see complex training in week 5.

PRINCIPLE #4 DROP SETS

Drop sets increase the volume of your workout by having you extend your sets beyond when you'd typically stop. The drop refers to performing an exercise and then reducing the weight by 20 to 30 percent, and immediately performing another set of the same exercise. For example, if you were doing deadlifts, you would perform a set with the prescribed weight. Then you'd immediately remove 20 to 30 percent of the weight and complete another set. This strength-to-speed contrast allows you to emphasize speed of movement on the dropped set and thus complete more reps, challenge your muscle further, and ignite your metabolism. I love drop sets! You'll begin to see drop sets in week 6.

PRINCIPLE #5 ECCENTRIC TRAINING

In week 7, you'll be introduced to eccentric training. This technique has commonly been referred to as "negatives" because you lower the weight slowly during the negative—or lowering—portion of the movement. I've decided not to use the term negative, because there is nothing negative about this very positive type of training. We'll call it by its scientific name: eccentric training.

When doing eccentric training, you are approximately 120 percent stronger in the eccentric (lowering) phase than in the lifting phase because your muscles can oppose more force than they can generate. It is easier to lower the weight slowly during a bench press (you are resisting or opposing the force of the weight) than it is to press it up off your chest quickly (generating power by pushing).

Besides allowing you to use more weight, focusing on the eccentric portion of an exercise actually leads to more muscle growth. That's because your muscles elongate during the eccentric (lowering) portion of the exercise, which causes more muscle recruitment. You should take 4 to 6 seconds to lower the weight, depending on the movement, and have a spotter assist you back to the starting position. You will typically decrease your reps and increase your weight when performing eccentric reps. Eccentric training is a great way to overcome plateaus and increase your overall strength.

THE IMPACT EQUIPMENT

Simple, effective, inexpensive— the only pieces of fitness equipment you need to transform your body.

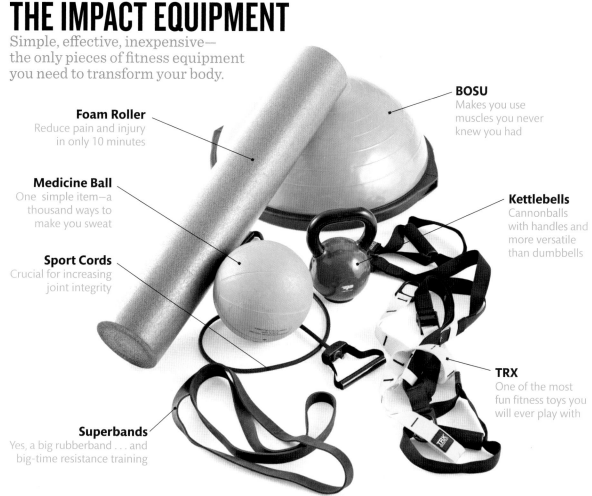

Foam Roller
Reduce pain and injury in only 10 minutes

Medicine Ball
One simple item—a thousand ways to make you sweat

Sport Cords
Crucial for increasing joint integrity

Superbands
Yes, a big rubberband . . . and big-time resistance training

BOSU
Makes you use muscles you never knew you had

Kettlebells
Cannonballs with handles and more versatile than dumbbells

TRX
One of the most fun fitness toys you will ever play with

The Muscle Matrix
Part Three

||||||||||||||||||||||||||||||||||||||||||||||||||||||||||||||||

GAME-CHANGING EQUIPMENT FOR BUILDING A HIGH-PERFORMANCE BODY

You've seen most of what makes the Muscle Matrix unique, but there's one last piece that'll have you working at an all-pro level. The equipment you'll use strays from that of typical workouts. You may even be using pieces of equipment you've never heard of or seen before. But don't worry. They aren't expensive. Most progressive gyms and training studios will have the majority of what I'd like you to use. Even if they had nothing, you could still build your own home gym from scratch for $250 to $500 and do every single exercise in this program. Or you could use some of my alternative exercises (page 270) and invest less. Either way, it's time to reinvent your training environment and make sure you have all the tools necessary for the IMPACT program.

TRX Suspension Training

Walk into my facility, Fitness Quest 10, and one thing catches your eye immediately. Almost every workout includes exercises suspended from long black and yellow nylon straps with handles and foot cradles on the ends of them. This is the TRX, a versatile and portable performance training tool

THE WORLD'S BIGGEST *fitness myths* 7

I need machines to get a total workout.

Nonsense. This is antiquated thinking. It certainly seems true, though—what do you see when you walk into almost every gym in the country? Machines. But machines lock you into an inflexible range of motion, one that does not mimic real, functional movement. They don't take into account your body type or height. They don't engage smaller stabilizing muscles the way free weights or the recommended IMPACT equipment does. IMPACT trains you for real-world movement and real-world strength, which will deliver what you really want—real-world results!

What Is Suspension Training? /// Suspension training positions your body so it works harder against the forces of gravity. It allows for maximum recruitment of muscle fibers and helps with overall strength, joint integrity, and core conditioning to build muscular balance. Suspension training is useful for everyone, because it utilizes your body weight as its main form of resistance. By simply adjusting your position, you can make each exercise easier or more challenging.

---

that uses your body weight as the only resistance you need for a complete workout. (The TRX creates an unstable training environment that allows you to work your small stabilizing muscles.) Plus, the whole unit rolls up, weighs only 2 pounds, and is easy to travel with, so you never have an excuse not to train.

Superbands

Superbands don't look like much. But these light, large rubber bands can be used for dozens of multidirectional exercises, add resistance to almost any exercise, or assist with movements such as pullups or chinups. But you'll also experience a huge difference when you use Superbands for your core work. You'll challenge your abs like never before. For men, I'd recommend the 1-inch or $1^3/_4$-inch bands. For women, go with the $^1/_2$-inch or 1-inch bands. And just like the TRX, Superbands can be easily tucked away in your suitcase for fitness on the go. I travel with Superbands and my TRX all the time.

Sport Cords

Meet the Superbands' little brother. Sport Cords serve the same purpose as the large rubber bands, only this version uses tubing that offers less resistance. This makes Sport Cords perfect for your joint integrity work, such as protecting the small muscles in your shoulders and rotator cuffs. Or, if you're building up your strength, you can substitute Sport Cords for exercises done with Superbands. While they may offer less resistance than Superbands, these tubes are not reserved just for women. Fellas, there are multiple Sport Cord exercises you can do to really work your body in unique ways.

Kettlebells

These "cannonballs with handles" have several unique characteristics that will enhance your training. The handle actually improves your grip

I've been fortunate to coach dozens of NFL quarterbacks and Major League pitchers—athletes who rely on their shoulders for their supper—and the lessons I've learned working with them can apply to you.

Most shoulder injuries to "overhead" athletes (quarterbacks, pitchers, volleyball players, tennis players) occur in the deceleration phase of throwing, or when you're slowing down the speed of your arm after you make contact or release a ball from your hand. Weekend warriors and recreational athletes are especially vulnerable to this because of a problem known as upper-crossed syndrome. This results when your chest and front-side shoulder muscles are too tight and end up rounding forward. You can easily identify this problem if you look at your profile in a mirror. This structural shift in your shoulders can end up eventually straining your rotator cuffs and leading to significant injuries that either limit your training abilities or land you on the operating table.

The shoulder integrity routine you'll perform with Sport Cords—included in the Joint Integrity portion of the IMPACT workouts in the back of the book—does an excellent job improving your posture, warming up your shoulders for heavier lifts such as the bench press, and helping establish muscle balance between the front side and back side of your body. Because the back side of your shoulders is often neglected, this aspect of the IMPACT program is vital to prevent injury and boost your performance.

strength, which has been linked to total-body performance. When you grip an object, it sends a signal to your brain to activate your muscles. The stronger your grip, the better the neurochemical signal, which allows you to activate more muscle fibers and lift more weight. Even better: Some research has linked strong grip strength to a longer life span. Which makes sense—after all, a powerful grip is associated with strength, fitness, and overall health.

The unique kettlebell design also allows for greater range of motion in your muscles, and diverse exercises that incorporate strength, speed, power, and core strength.

BOSU Ball

Way back in 1999, my colleague David Weck created the BOSU ball. I had one of the first prototypes, and the tool—with its half-dome, half-platform appearance—looked like some Swiss-ball science experiment. But once I tried it, it became a staple of all my programming. The BOSU creates instability in a safe way that increases the difficulty of any core, balance, or strength and conditioning exercise. You'll love the diversity and challenge a BOSU offers.

Foam Roller

As you learned in Chapter 4, "Secrets to a Pain-Free Body," these firm, foam-packed rollers allow you to perform self-massage (self-myofascial release),

TONY GWYNN JR.
OUTFIELDER
SAN DIEGO PADRES

Todd Durkin client for 1 year

WHY HE NEEDS IMPACT TRAINING: "My training background has always come from football, so I really needed intensity. And man, on day one, intensity is what I got!"

WHEN HE REALIZED IMPACT MADE A DIFFERENCE: "Inside of 2 months I noticed a huge difference in a) how my body felt and the strength I was gaining without lifting a whole bunch of weights, and b) when I started to run. My explosiveness was a lot better than it had been in the past. And my wheels are a big part of my game."

HIS TRAINING SECRET: "I'll go back to intensity. If you're not training with intensity every time, you're not getting as much out the workout as you can. Go hard and get after it."

The Power of the BOSU /// When I first worked with Drew Brees in 2003, his weakest area was his core. I remember we were doing BOSU sideups (an exercise you'll find in this program), and we did 15 reps and then held the final rep for barely 30 seconds. After just 1 set, Drew's obliques were reeling in pain. It showed me that even though he was an NFL quarterback, he had a long way to go to improve his body. He made up that ground—and then some! The off-season before Drew led the Saints to a victory in Super Bowl XLIV (44), he routinely ended his workouts with 44 reps of this exercise and then held it for another 44 seconds. That truly is world class!

which improves your fascia. Foam rolling is a great way to prevent injury or rid your body of aches and pains that you may be experiencing. But I'll warn you: This isn't a soothing experience. When you foam roll over soft tissue, it's often tender, sensitive, or even painful. That just means your soft tissue is not healthy and needs to be worked. All my athletes and clients start their workouts with foam rolling for 5 to 10 minutes, and they also do it at home. I recommend you do the same. Remember, if you don't like it, that means you need it! Foam rolling is the poor man's version of getting a massage every day. And we would all love that, right?

Tennis Balls

Tennis balls are a great tool for self-massage, much like a foam roller, but for the bottoms of your feet. The plantar aponeurosis, a $1/2$-inch-thick band of fascia lining the sole of your foot from heel to toes, plays a critical role in your posture, in injury prevention, and in your kinetic chain. And a tennis ball can work this area. Bad feet can wreak havoc on your knees, back, and entire body, so this exercise can pay huge dividends.

Barbells and Dumbbells

Most exercise programs use barbells and dumbbells, and the workouts you'll do in this book are no exception. Both of these pieces of equipment are found at every gym and offer a wide variety of exercises that you can perform. What you might not know is that free weights, such as barbells and dumbbells, challenge your body more than machines do, according to a study in the *Journal of Strength and Conditioning Research.* Not only do they increase muscle activation, but they also increase range of motion and are less likely to cause injury. In the IMPACT program, you'll see traditional exercises, such as bench presses and lunges, but you'll also learn many unique, new movements that will maximally challenge your body and bring fun back into your workouts.

Folks, you just had a master class in advanced fitness techniques. Now it's time to see how you'll put all this new knowledge to good use. It's also time to see exactly what you're in for. . . .

---

11 Great Stretches to IMPACT Your Flexibility /// See page 266.

1 SB Chest Stretch
2 Kneeling Hip Flexor Stretch
3 Cat & Dog
4 Downward Dog
5 Upward Dog
6 Pigeon Pose
7 Figure 4 Stretch
8 SB Hamstring Stretch
9 SB Groin Stretch
10 SB Lower Back Stretch
11 SB Side-Lying Quad/
  Hip Flexor Stretch

6
YOUR
GAME PLAN

 "Great moments are born from great opportunities."
— HERB BROOKS

Now that you know how the Muscle Matrix works, it's time to put it into action. Your 10-week transformation consists of three stages. Each will be color coded in the workout section of this book, so you can easily identify where you are in the program. Training Camp (Stage I) will be marked by the color green, In Season (Stage II) will be blue, and The Playoffs (Stage III) will be red. Remember, the workouts are designed to increase in difficulty as you advance. But it's essential that you follow the program as it's designed, including performing all seven phases of the Muscle Matrix. Don't worry if you don't have some of the equipment yet. I've created a list of alternatives that will train your body in similar movements. Obviously, the equipment I've suggested is ideal, but you can still reach all your goals using the alternative options.

Stage I
Training Camp
WEEKS 1, 2, AND 3

This 3-week break-in period will allow you to experience and master the fundamentals of the Muscle Matrix. During Training Camp, you'll complete three total-body workouts and one boot camp workout per week. Each training day is followed by a day off from resistance training, when you can either rest and recover or perform your preferred form of movement activity, such as traditional steady-state cardio, cycling, or playing a sport.

The goals of this first stage are simple but essential to your ultimate success. Your muscles and cardiovascular system will be challenged, of course, but you're also using this time to master new exercises you may never have tried before. The most difficult adjustment will probably be tempo. I want you to get to a point where you're never resting more than 1 minute after a set or exercise. You will most likely be sucking wind throughout your IMPACT workouts. This is good. As I've always said, you need to "get breathless" every day. But if you ever feel nauseated or dizzy, slow down or stop. Otherwise, it's time to enjoy the fruits of your labor and get after it!

Like every workout in this regimen, your program starts with foam rolling and the dynamic warmup. Ideally, you'll perform this warmup routine on every training day, as it sets the tone for a great workout every time. During your 3-week Training Camp, you'll be activating your entire neuromuscular system and building the foundation for better movement through joint integrity and core conditioning. You will improve your flexibility, build strength, and improve rhythm and coordination, while becoming familiar with the demands of high-intensity interval training. You'll also begin to train with the TRX and learn the new demands it will place on your body. By the end of your break-in program, you should experience total-body changes, feel stronger, move better, and start to truly understand the challenges and benefits of this program.

Deciphering the Matrix

The total-body workouts you'll perform in the first stage of IMPACT will most likely be different from what you're used to. Each workout can be divided

---

Important notes /// IMPACT calls for 4 or 5 days of training per week, depending on the stage of the plan. You can do an extra 1 or 2 days of cardio each week if you would like. If you can't be outdoors due to inclement weather, you can do the same type of body-weight interval-style training in the gym or in your home as you combine cardio and resistance training. Your cardio could be jumping rope or using any machine that you prefer, such as a treadmill or elliptical trainer.

---

into four separate circuits. The first three circuits each consist of three exercises that you'll perform back-to-back with only 30 to 60 seconds of rest between moves. You'll combine a lower-body exercise and two upper-body exercises in each of the circuits. One upper-body exercise will focus on a push (such as a pushup or bench press), while the other will utilize a pulling motion (such as a row or pullup). This offers a balanced approach to challenging all the muscles in your body.

Within those three circuits, you'll equally work your upper and lower body and the front-side and back-side muscles, and also work on single-arm and single-leg exercises, which ensures that you won't build any muscle imbalances. The final two-exercise circuit provides auxiliary work by targeting smaller muscle groups and special-emphasis training. You'll rotate among working on your arms, your shoulders, and balance. It looks like this:

CIRCUIT 1	CIRCUIT 2	CIRCUIT 3	CIRCUIT 4
1a Lower body	**2a** Lower body	**3a** Lower body single leg	**4a** Auxiliary work
1b Upper body push	**2b** Upper body push	**3b** Upper body single arm; push	**4b** Auxiliary work
1c Upper body pull	**2c** Upper body pull	**3c** Upper body single arm; pull	

Cardio burns the most fat.

Not true. Resistance training burns the most calories overall. When you do cardio, you're burning calories during the activity. With resistance training, you burn calories during the activity but keep burning them for up to 48 hours afterward. This is known as excess postexercise oxygen consumption (EPOC), or the more well-known afterburn. Resistance training also jacks up your metabolism, improves insulin resistance, and shuts down the fat-storing enzymes in your body.

Don't misunderstand me: I love cardio, and it's a part of this plan. Remember, cardio is just another form of movement, which is one of the seven basic principles of the Muscle Matrix. Exercise is never a bad thing, but make sure you add variety. Some days you can go for a long, slow run, while other days you can run sprints to accelerate your results. Pickup basketball and soccer are always great. And don't forget the cardio benefits of games like racquetball, handball, beach volleyball, and ultimate Frisbee! Just understand that cardio by itself is not the most efficient way to burn calories and fat. No one will look his or her best without resistance training, a cornerstone of the IMPACT program.

"Nobody ever drowned in sweat!"
— JACK "BEAR" ROBERTS, BRICK HIGH SCHOOL (NEW JERSEY) FOOTBALL TRAINER

Stage II
In Season
WEEKS 4, 5, 6, AND 7

Once your body has adjusted to the demands of the program, you'll advance to the next stage of your transformation. You'll master different Matrix principles that maximize the effect of every exercise, including plyometrics, complex sets, drop sets, and eccentric training.

This will start in week 4 with plyometrics, in which you'll learn how to build explosive power and move more effortlessly in everyday living. You'll then progress to complex sets, which take high-intensity interval training to the next level: You'll pair a weighted exercise with a body-weight movement to build explosiveness and provide a boost to your metabolism. From there, you'll do drop sets in week 6, which will bump up your exercise volume, jolt your muscles by allowing you to perform more work in less time, and require mental and physical strength to help you push yourself to new heights.

This Matrix sequence ends with eccentric training, in which we manipulate the amount of time that your muscles remain under tension by making reps last longer. As I described in Chapter 4, we do this by slowing down the lowering portion of specific exercises. Not only will this allow your body to handle heavier loads than normal, but it's also an excellent way to overcome plateaus and build more strength.

Split Fusion Training

This 4-week stage also blends a unique form of split fusion workouts. Instead of total-body workouts three times a week, you'll mix full-body plans with individual upper- and lower-body workouts. This allows you to add more volume. Additionally,

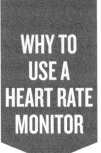

WHY TO USE A HEART RATE MONITOR

I love heart rate monitors. They show you how hard you're training, and they can track how many calories you've burned during your workout—and I find it incredibly motivating to see how many calories I've torched during a session. If your intensity is right, it's not uncommon for men to burn 600 to 800 calories and women to burn 500 to 700 calories during an IMPACT workout. This calorie burn is typically based on gender, metabolism, total duration of the workout, and, of course, intensity. During a boot camp workout, it's common for a man to burn between 800 and 1,200 calories and a woman to burn 600 to 800 calories. Burn, baby, burn! I encourage you to keep your training intensity elevated to 65 to 85 percent of your maximum heart rate for at least 30 minutes of each training session.

it allows more rest between training sessions for the same muscle group and helps prevent overtraining as your volume increases.

Each week ends with an innovative Saturday body-weight boot camp, which ignites your metabolism to burn fat faster and leaves you ready to enjoy the weekend. It also gets you outside (hopefully!) to play and enjoy the great outdoors. If you have the cardio bug, you can add 1 or 2 days of the cardio of your choice per week, but make sure your body is not breaking down and is recovering well, and that you feel great. You should take at least 1 day, and preferably 2, of complete rest each week.

Calculate your target heart rate using the Karvonen Formula:

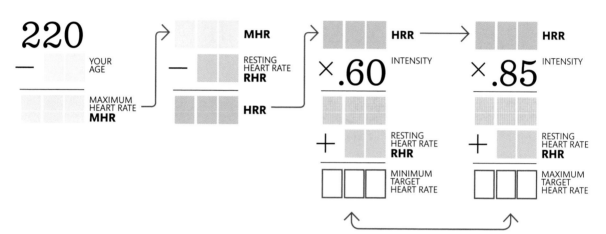

STEP 1	STEP 2	STEP 3	STEP 4
Calculate your **Maximum Heart Rate (MHR)**	Calculate your **Heart Rate Reserve (HRR)**	Determine your **minimum target heart rate** during exercise	Determine your **maximum target heart rate** during exercise

220
— YOUR AGE
MAXIMUM HEART RATE **MHR**

— MHR
RESTING HEART RATE **RHR**
HRR

HRR
× .60 INTENSITY
RESTING HEART RATE **RHR**
+ MINIMUM TARGET HEART RATE

HRR
× .85 INTENSITY
RESTING HEART RATE **RHR**
+ MAXIMUM TARGET HEART RATE

Your heart rate should be between the minimum and maximum beats per minute when training.

Split Fusion looks like this:

MONDAY	WEDNESDAY	THURSDAY	SATURDAY
1a Total body	**2a** Upper body	**3a** Lower body and Core	**4a** Total body boot camp

IMPACT Training: "In Season" Programming

WEEK 4: Plyometrics

WEEK 5: Complexes

WEEK 6: Drop sets

WEEK 7: Eccentric training

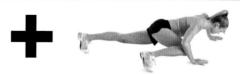

Upgrade the Dynamic Warmup /// During Stage II of the program, you'll slightly adjust the dynamic warmup phase of the Muscle Matrix. You'll still complete the 15 original exercises, but you'll also add a new movement: lizard crawls. This fun yet challenging movement combines a crawling motion with a pushup and will help prepare your upper body and core for your upcoming workout. Include lizard crawls as part of your warmup for the rest of the program.

Stage III
The Playoffs
WEEKS 8, 9, AND 10

Seven weeks in, you'll have witnessed a dramatic transformation. By this point, if you are following the World-Class Eating program (coming in Chapter 8) and focusing on additional recovery and regeneration strategies (coming in Chapter 9), you will have lost pounds of fat, seen muscle on your body like never before, fit into clothes you thought you'd have to throw out, begun to feel more energetic, developed more confidence, and become fired up for the final 3-week stage of the program . . . The Playoffs!

Now it's time to turn up the heat. The final 3 weeks is fun. Put it all together and get ready for your own personal Super Bowl run. Your result will be a transformation that truly is world class.

After learning and implementing new strategies designed to challenge your body to lose fat and build lean muscle, you'll enter the final stage of the program, where everything comes together. You'll be training at a high level and incorporating every component of the Matrix, from the seven phases to the advanced training techniques, and every piece of equipment. Some portions may seem very difficult, but your body and mind will be prepared to pass the challenge. And through it all, remember that this entire program was designed to have you "play," to get back to running, jumping, lifting, moving, throwing. And smiling. The workouts should be enjoyable and one of the best parts of your day. After all 10 weeks, you should be looking and feeling your best.

At the end of this program, you should feel like a new person. More energy, more confidence, less stress. Proud owner of a completely remade body.

IMPACT SECRETS
from the pros

CHARLES TILLMAN
CORNERBACK
CHICAGO BEARS

Todd Durkin client for 3 years

WHY HE NEEDS IMPACT TRAINING: "I've had back and shoulder surgeries, so I needed to expand my entire training mindset to make sure I can stay healthy and still play at the highest level. Without this training, I wouldn't be playing as well as I am."

WHEN HE REALIZED IMPACT MADE A DIFFERENCE:
"When I walked into TD's gym and saw the book *212°* sitting there at the front desk. I love that book, and it turns out TD does, too, so I knew we had the exact same mindset when it comes to training—push 1 degree harder every time. At 211 degrees, water's hot. At 212 degrees, it boils. Boiling water makes steam, and steam can move a locomotive. Go get that extra degree. There's always something more you can do, an extra set, an extra rep. That 1 degree makes all the difference."

HIS TRAINING SECRET: "Open your mind to different activities you've never tried. This year is my first doing Pilates. I hate it but I love it, you know what I mean? It was the biggest thing I could do to help myself prolong my career. It helps my flexibility, shoulders, and core strength. I see a huge difference in my hips. I could never sit Indian-style before. Now I'm like, 'Hey, I can sit Indian-style.' I've been loosened up in ways I didn't think were possible."

But your transformation isn't complete. First, I want you to throttle down for a couple of days. You've earned it! You'll want the rest, because One Big Challenge still awaits. On the Saturday of your 10th week on the program, you're going to perform the eight exercises you first completed in the self-test section of the book (coming in Chapter 7). That's right. Post-test time. Do everything all over again, and then compare it with where you were 10 weeks ago. You'll see how dramatically your performance has changed in only 10 weeks. You should be faster, stronger, and better conditioned, and you should have improved on your weaknesses. Exercises that were once difficult should be easier, and the entire self-test should feel different to your body. You'll be shocked to see the new person you've become. And the changes won't just be skin deep. You'll feel better, smile more, live healthier. And you'll realize that you can make the types of changes you once thought impossible. That's IMPACT, baby!

CAN YOU TRAIN TOO HARD?

The IMPACT workouts in this program are designed to challenge your body harder than you're used to. But it's important to make sure that you're not pushing your body too much. Overtraining occurs when you do a poor job of allowing your body to adapt to your routine and don't prioritize your recovery and regeneration (which you'll learn about in the next two chapters). Soreness is a result of working hard, so that doesn't mean you're overtraining. But keep an eye out for the following symptoms:

▶ Increase in resting heart rate and blood pressure
▶ Decrease in performance
▶ Trouble sleeping
▶ Stomach problems
▶ Consistent low energy and bad mood

If you experience several of these for a sustained period of time, scale back on your exercise. And when you return, make sure you apply all the tips provided in the nutrition and sleep, recovery, and regeneration chapters to help keep your body healthy.

"Never, never, never give up."

— WINSTON CHURCHILL

7
THE IMPACT FIT TEST

 "You are as strong as your weakest link . . . and as efficient as your worst movement."

—TOM HOUSE, PITCHING COACH, NATIONAL PITCHING ASSOCIATION

When LaDainian Tomlinson first started

working with me in 2002, he was fast, strong, agile, and flexible—all the traits you want in a great running back. If I'd have run him through the gauntlet of typical NFL tests, like the bench press, 40-yard dash, or shuttle runs, he'd have passed with flying colors. But LaDainian wasn't looking for a pat on the back or reassurance of his abilities. He wanted to get better, and he needed a starting point. That's what happens when you want to be best in class. You're not afraid to start from ground zero and work your way up.

Instead of having him do the same thing as everyone else, I tested him on exercises that would reveal potential weaknesses. This was essential, because it would provide a baseline that we could use to gauge his improvement. I wanted to see how LaDainian moved doing simple exercises, knowing that these tests would reveal plenty about his performance. After a dynamic warmup, his first test was a single-leg balance touch. It requires you to stand on one leg, bend at your hips while keeping your back flat, touch the floor, and then stand all the way back up. You have to touch the floor as many times as possible in 60 seconds.

The first time LaDainian tried the test, he was able to touch the floor 32 times on his right leg but only 23 times on his left. Aha! Weakness found. A lightbulb went on, and LaDainian saw how a simple test of movement could potentially reap huge rewards in his performance. While he was frustrated at his physical imbalances, he was excited to fix his shortcomings and improve his performance.

Now I want to test you. Here's a series of exercises that you can do yourself that will reveal your basic fitness level. You will complete this test to start week 1 and repeat it at the end of week 10. Think pre-test and post-test. You can't measure progress without a baseline. And that's what makes a self-test so important before you start a program. Although your ultimate success won't be measured in yards or touchdowns, I'd love for you to have a baseline against which to measure your improvements during the course of this program and beyond.

There are a total of eight exercises in this self-test. Two exercises are subjective and six are objective. This is not as much a formal assessment (for that you'll need something like the Functional Movement Screen—see the box at the right) as it is a snapshot of where you are now. The first two exercises will show how well you move. You might not realize that your body is tight in certain areas or that you have a limited range of motion. These exercises are eye-openers that will show you how much you need to work on your fascia and improve your stability and mobility.

The second stage of the self-test is a six-exercise challenge that will act as your fitness baseline and give you an idea of your strength, endurance, conditioning, core strength, and balance capabilities. You may do well, or you might struggle. It doesn't matter. What does matter is how you improve over

and then some
FUNCTIONAL MOVEMENT SCREEN

The Functional Movement Screen is a full-body assessment composed of seven fundamental movement patterns that require a balance of mobility and stability. You score 1, 2, or 3 on each movement pattern, for a possible maximum score of 21. Most people score between 14 and 16 points. The test places your body in positions in which weaknesses and imbalances become noticeable. From there, you're able to identify flawed movement patterns, and then you can develop an exercise program around improving your movements and making yourself more efficient in all activities. If you want more information on the Functional Movement Screen, visit www.functionalmovement.com. You do require a skilled practitioner to conduct this screen.

time. If you follow all the steps I provide in this book, including the workouts, nutrition, and recovery and regeneration recommendations, I know you will see dramatic improvements. If you truly focus on becoming 1 percent better every day, just think how great you'll be after 10 weeks.

If you feel pain /// These tests are designed to assess your current fitness level. However, if at any time you find that any of these movements causes you pain (which is not to be confused with fatigue), I advise you to see a physician or physical therapist to make sure that there's no underlying injury requiring professional attention.

The IMPACT Fit Test

Perform the exercises below in the order listed. Rest for 2 to 3 minutes after each exercise to make sure that you're not fatigued for the next one. Do this routine before you start the first week of the IMPACT workout. You'll repeat the same exercises at the end of the 10-week program to see how much you've improved.

EXERCISE	PRE-TEST *Week 1*	POST-TEST *Week 10*
Overhead squat *10 reps*	NOTES	NOTES
Wall slide *10 reps*	NOTES	NOTES
Hover plank *max time*	TIME	TIME
Deadlift *5 reps with max weight*	WEIGHT	WEIGHT
Pushup *as many reps as possible in 60 seconds*	REPS	REPS
Single-leg balance touch *as many reps as possible in 60 seconds*	REPS RIGHT LEG LEFT LEG	REPS RIGHT LEG LEFT LEG
Rack row *as many reps as possible in 60 seconds*	REPS	REPS
300-yard shuttle run *as fast as you can run*	TIME	TIME

▶ OVERHEAD SQUAT

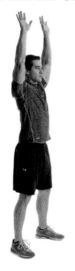
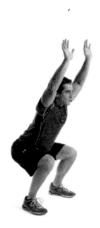

Stand with your feet shoulder-width apart and fully extend your arms above your head, slightly wider than shoulder-width apart. Lower your body as far as you can by pushing your hips back and bending your knees. Your torso should stay as upright as possible. Pause, then slowly push yourself back to the starting position. Perform 10 repetitions.

WHAT IT TELLS YOU: Watching yourself in a mirror helps answer the following questions:

• Can you lower your body until your thighs are below parallel to the floor? (Are your knees bent past 90 degrees?)

• Can you keep your heels on the floor?

• Can you keep your toes pointing straight ahead?

• Can your hands stay above your head as you squat, and your back and chest remain in a neutral position (and not lean forward)?

• Do your knees stay in place and not cave inward?

If you don't answer yes to all of these questions, it could mean a variety of weaknesses, ranging from poor mobility in your upper and lower body to poor stabilization and control.

▶ WALL SLIDE

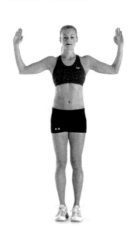
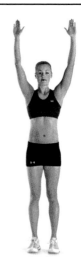

Stand with your butt, upper back, and head against a wall. Place your hands and arms against the wall in the "high-five" position, elbows bent 90 degrees and upper arms at shoulder height. Keeping your elbows, wrists, and hands against the wall, slide your elbows down toward your sides as far as you can. Squeeze your shoulder blades together as you go. Then slide your arms back up the wall as high as you can while keeping your hands in contact with the wall. Complete 10 reps.

WHAT IT TELLS YOU: Your movement pattern and how your body feels during this exercise can tell you a lot about your upper body.

• Do your elbows or hands come off the wall?

• How high can you slide your hands up the wall? Can you get them overhead?

• Do you feel any pain in your shoulders or upper back?

• Can you keep your shoulder blades squeezed together?

If you struggle with this exercise, it probably means you need to improve your scapular/midthoracic mobility and the flexibility of your chest and shoulder region. Otherwise, you are too tight on the front side of your body, and you're placing your body at risk of injury, especially when you do any pressing exercises, such as the bench press.

▶ HOVER PLANK | p. 228

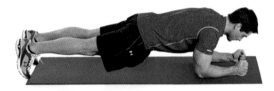

Set a stopwatch and perform a plank for as long as you can.

WHAT IT TELLS YOU: This test assesses your core strength, including that of your abs, lower back, and glutes. Improving your core strength and endurance will be extremely important to your success in almost every exercise you'll do in the IMPACT workout.

▶ BARBELL DEADLIFT | p. 266

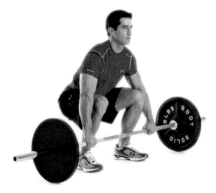

After a thorough warmup, select the heaviest weight that you can lift for 5 repetitions.

WHAT IT TELLS YOU: The deadlift is one of the best exercises for assessing total-body strength. Whether you're a man or a woman, you want your body to be able to move efficiently. The deadlift mimics picking an object off the floor, which is one of the most common daily movements.

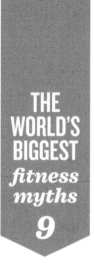

THE WORLD'S BIGGEST *fitness myths* 9

I'm too out of shape for this program.

No, you're not. You're ready for it, no matter who you are. The IMPACT program is designed to adapt to anyone at any fitness level. Here's why: The beginning of the program is based primarily on body-weight training, which means it's not about moving a lot of iron. You'll also use "intuitive training," meaning you'll listen to your body, ramp up when you feel strong, and dial it back when you feel weak.

I've said before that my clientele is a collection of people just like anyone else: middle-aged executives, grandparents, homemakers, 40-year-old deconditioned weekend warriors, you name it, I've got 'em. They all do this program, they all have a blast, and they all see results. You will, too.

PUSHUP | p. 229

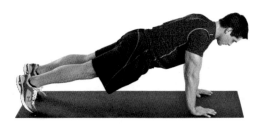

Do as many pushups as you can in 1 minute.
WHAT IT TELLS YOU: Pushups are a great assessment of upper-body strength and conditioning. They also rely on core strength and shoulder mobility, which will both be improved in the program. Note: If you pre-test doing modified pushups from the knees, you should post-test the same way.

SINGLE-LEG BALANCE TOUCH | p. 225

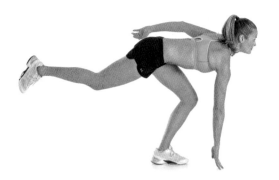

Set a timer for 60 seconds, stand on your left leg, and perform as many balance touches as you can in 60 seconds. Keep your left knee slightly bent and your back flat, and be sure to reach down and touch the floor. If you lose your balance and mess up, regain your balance and keep going. Record your

cumulative score after 60 seconds. Then repeat the process on your right leg.
WHAT IT TELLS YOU: This is a great test of your balance and whether you have any strength imbalances between your two sides. One of the best ways to build a better body is to eliminate any imbalances that exist—the IMPACT program will help.

RACK ROW | p. 235

Complete as many rows as you can in 60 seconds.
WHAT IT TELLS YOU: Much like pushups, rows provide an assessment of upper-body strength and conditioning. But unlike pushups, this exercise measures the often-neglected muscles on the back side of your body.

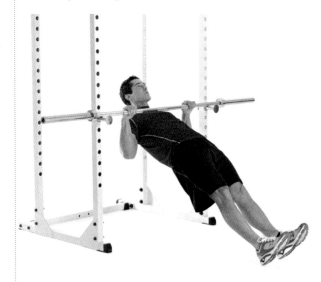

▶ 300-YARD SHUTTLE RUN

Mark off a 25-yard distance. Run the 25 yards, then run back to where you started. Complete this 50-yard round-trip run 6 times and record your time.

WHAT IT TELLS YOU: It's a marker for speed and conditioning. A world-class time is anything less than 60 seconds. (The best I've ever seen is 52 seconds.) It doesn't really matter what your time is the first time you test. What matters most is that you improve your time the next time you're tested.

Congratulations! You've just given yourself a crucial set of statistics that you'll use as the baseline of your fitness for the next 10 weeks. As I've said, these are not pass-or-fail tests. They're great fitness markers, and when you retake these same eight tests after you finish the IMPACT program, you will see inspiring, even eye-popping evidence of your transformation. I'm not exaggerating. In this game, it ain't whether you win or lose, but how much you improve, and I believe in my heart that your total fitness improvement will surpass your expectations. Savor the flavor, my friend, because you'll have earned it!

And, speaking of flavor, are you hungry? I hope so. Because the next chapter delivers World-Class Eating, the IMPACT nutrition plan that will provide the launching pad for great workouts and amazing results—fuel for your fire, baby. Let's eat!

IMPACT SECRETS *from the pros*

TIM STAUFFER

PITCHER
SAN DIEGO PADRES

Todd Durkin client for 1 year

WHY HE NEEDS IMPACT TRAINING: "Improving my core strength was the biggest thing for me going in. And I definitely did that. Players always say this, but I literally wanted to go into Spring Training in the best shape of my life. I wanted to be able to keep a certain intensity level all year on the field and I needed these workouts to make a difference.

"You feel more athletic doing TD's workouts with all the different movements, constant motion, not just always laying on a bench pushing up dumbbells. There was always a specific reason why we were doing what we were doing."

WHEN HE REALIZED IMPACT MADE A DIFFERENCE: "I noticed going into Spring Training. I felt different. Stronger, better conditioned, and especially in how quickly I recovered from the everyday grind of baseball. And looking back, the workouts helped me win a job."

HIS TRAINING SECRET: "Two things. First, work out with friends. It was a lot easier working out with a group of guys I play with. It formed a bigger bond than we would have just playing during the season. You become a tighter group going through workouts together. And you can get some friendly competition going, which makes you work harder and not even know it. And second, if you're looking for a trainer, don't just go with the first person you meet. Having access to someone with such knowledge in sports training and who knows how to get a body prepared is a huge advantage. I'm fortunate to have access to TD and all of his knowledge."

8
WORLD-CLASS EATING

 "Let your food be your medicine and your medicine be your food."

—HIPPOCRATES

It's time to "get your mind right" about food.

Our country has an eating problem. Along with high stress and a sedentary lifestyle, poor eating habits have led our country into a frightening new reality. Heart disease, stroke, cancer, and diabetes tear at the roots of our health because we aren't willing to make the necessary changes in our lives. And despite technological advances and improvements in health care, we're worse off than ever. More people are overweight or obese than at any time in recorded history. The childhood obesity epidemic has grown at an alarming rate. It's so bad that this current generation of children is expected to have a shorter life span than their parents. Why? Because we don't exercise enough and we don't eat right. (Check out the sidebar on metabolic syndrome to see what I mean.)

But the more important question is, what are we going to do about it?

First, we must change how we think about food.

Instead of seeing food as essential fuel for our bodies, most of us think of it as a reward or a comfort. For some people, food is very much a drug. You eat to feel good. You chow down to cheer up, and turn to bad foods to deal with stress. When you celebrate success, you go out for a big meal. When you're dragging or you've had a rough day, you often drown your feelings in comfort food or alcohol to satisfy your emotions temporarily. How healthy is that?

When I told you earlier to get your mind right, it applied to everything you do. Too many people don't realize that the food they're putting in their bodies may be toxic. Or they just aren't willing to make the change until something bad happens.

Change isn't easy, but it can be simple. The guidelines you'll follow in this program are simple. After all, I love the basics. Food is fuel, and fuel is energy. Without fuel in your automobile, your car would sputter, struggle, and eventually stop running. Your body is no different. Put the wrong foods—or no food at all—in your system and you'll struggle. Putter and come to a stop. Collapse. Maybe even die.

The changes I'm going to suggest are very doable, if you are willing to change. This is about nutritious, delicious, healthful eating. I'll teach you the why, when, what, and how of the IMPACT nutrition plan. Humans are naturally energetic beings, after all. You'll be amazed how you feel and perform when you have the right grade of gas in your tank.

Let's get started!

On this plan, you're going to eat—and eat some more! But it's not about depending on just any food. I want you to eat the right types of foods that will provide energy for everything you do, and have you looking great. I love food. My wife, Melanie, is an excellent cook and prepares fantastic meals that I enjoy with my three kids. Food is one of the simplest pleasures in life. And right there is the key: simplicity. Simplicity will get your mind right about food. Instead of practicing avoidance and counting calories, I want you eating, savoring, and refueling by choosing the right foods.

Your New Nutrition Plan

I hope you're as fired up about this stage of the program as I am. The suggestions that follow deliver results. It's that simple. Have fun with this—you'll be experimenting and discovering new ways to fuel your body. Just remember, the key is changing slowly. Take one tip at a time, make the adjustments, and then add something new. Before you know it, you'll have transformed the way you eat, and that will unleash the kind of energy that will transform your life!

World-Class Eating is not a diet. It is a nutrition plan. Diets set us up for failure. Diets start and stop. Starting today, diets are over. World-Class Eating will teach you how to reinvent how you eat—not just for the better, but for the best!

THE 10 COMMANDMENTS OF IMPACT NUTRITION ///

IS METABOLIC SYNDROME KILLING YOU?

A big gut will most likely bring you an early death. That's because the larger your belly, the greater your risk of metabolic syndrome, a disastrous, degenerative body process that leads to the biggest killers facing society today: type-2 diabetes, heart disease, stroke, and cancer. If you tend to store fat in your gut—the "apple" body shape, as opposed to the "pear" body shape (in which more fat is carried on the hips)— your risk is higher. While men generally tend toward apple shapes, some women do as well.

HERE'S HOW METABOLIC SYNDROME WORKS:
When you overconsume foods that turn into glucose in your body (processed sugar, starches, and alcohol are the biggest culprits), your body can burn off only so much of the sweet stuff as energy, so your liver and pancreas work together to remove the rest or convert it to fat for storage. The pancreas pumps out the insulin needed to make this process happen. Some of this fat is stored in the liver itself. Some ends up in your bloodstream as triglycerides. Even more ends up as visceral fat, stored in and around the vital organs in your midsection. This belly fat is devastating, because the more you have, the more it inhibits the function of all these crucial organs. Meanwhile, as you continue to overconsume, your insulin can't do the redistribution job as efficiently or as effectively, because your body's insulin receptors lose their sensitivity from overwork; this is called insulin resistance. Your pancreas must pump out more and more insulin. You get fatter. Your receptors become more resistant, and this vicious cycle continues until your pancreas ultimately burns out. No more insulin! And you've gone from metabolic syndrome to full-blown type-2 diabetes.

The only cure for metabolic syndrome, and the best prevention for the health problems it brings on, is exercising, losing weight, eating better, and living a healthier lifestyle. No shortcuts!

First, visit your doctor and assess your general health. If you suffer from three or more of the following factors, you're at risk.

▶ Waist circumference greater than 40 inches (Measure across your belly button, not where your waistband rides.)
▶ HDL cholesterol (the good stuff) below 40 milligrams per deciliter
▶ Elevated triglycerides (higher than 150 milligrams per deciliter)
▶ Blood pressure higher than 115/75
▶ Fasting glucose above 100 milligrams per deciliter

---

1 **Get your motor started: Eat breakfast!**

2 **Slow down!**

3 **Fuel up before training.**

4 **Refuel after training.**

5 **Go wild!**

6 **Remember that supplements are just that—supplements!**

7 **Water your body.**

8 **Keep a nutrition journal.**

9 **Follow the 90-10 rule.**

10 **Experiment with the IMPACT menu.**

Preparation

The IMPACT nutrition plan provides an overview of how you should eat every day. I will give you essential information to help you plan your meals, eat out at restaurants, and aid your shopping experience. But, most important, I guarantee that you'll be preparing for success and powering up your body for maximum performance and optimal health. Use the following guidelines to streamline your decisions, and then check out a sample menu at the end of this chapter for more ideas.

Start ENJOYING

- Vegetables
- Fruits
- Brown rice
- Beans (not the baked variety)
- Hummus
- Whole grains (oatmeal, mullet, couscous, quinoa, sprouted grains)
- Raw nuts (almonds, cashews, pecans, walnuts)
- Natural butters (almond, cashew, macadamia, tahini, walnut)
- Oils (coconut, cold-pressed canola, extra-virgin olive, flax, sesame seed)
- Avocado
- Whole wheat pasta
- Wild coldwater fish (but avoid farm-raised)
- Eggs
- Whole grain breads and cereals
- Smart dairy choices (almond milk, feta cheese, Greek yogurt, etc.)
- Hormone-free, free-range turkey, chicken, and 100 percent grass-fed beef

Select these foods as frequently as possible as the basis for your meals. They offer the most nutrition and the best fuel for your body.

Stop CONSUMING

- Sugar (corn syrup, fructose, molasses, sucrose)
- Artificial sweeteners such as aspartame (NutraSweet, Equal), sucralose (Splenda), saccharin (Sweet'N Low), and acesulfame-K (Sunett)
- High-fructose corn syrup
- Fruit juices (fresh-squeezed is acceptable in moderation)
- Alcohol
- Soda
- Added salt
- White flour products
- White pasta
- White rice
- Fast food/fried food
- Soy-based products

The goal is clear. This is the list of foods to avoid. Period. If you need to, you can begin by identifying a goal and starting to cut back. Are you someone who drinks three diet sodas a day? Immediately reduce it to two. Next week reduce it to one. You get it. Challenge yourself to get 1 percent better every day. Soon you will have banished every one of these from the pantry and fridge. And your body.

Start DRINKING

- Half your body weight in fluid ounces of water daily
- Vegetable juice (fresh juiced)
- Green tea
- Herbal tea
- Coconut water / coconut milk
- Almond milk

IMPACT NUTRITION
in a Nutshell

||||||||||||||||||||||||||||||||||||||||||||||||||||||||||||||||||||||||||||||

▶ Eat three main meals and two or three snacks per day. Keep both the meals and the snacks small.

▶ Consume protein at every meal. Your goal is to eat 1 gram of protein per pound of your goal body weight (e.g., if you weigh 200 pounds and want to lose 30, shoot for 170 grams of protein daily). This may seem like a lot, but if you stick with high-quality, lean protein, it can help you reach your goals.

▶ Eat fresh produce as frequently as possible. Eating vegetables at almost every meal is one of the best ways to drop body fat fast.

▶ Don't avoid fats. They are essential—our bodies need them in order to function properly. Just eat the right kind of "good" fats, including nuts (such as almonds, cashews, and walnuts), avocado, olive oil, and nut butters.

▶ Your snacks should always include either a protein or a fat source.

▶ Before and after your workouts, combine carbohydrates and protein for optimal performance and recovery. Try blending a nutrient-filled protein shake (see "10 Tasty Protein Shake Recipes" on page 84) an hour before your IMPACT workout or within 30 minutes after a training session to aid in recovery.

IMPACT SECRETS *from* the pros

BEN LEBER
LINEBACKER
MINNESOTA VIKINGS

Todd Durkin client for 6 years

WHY HE NEEDS IMPACT TRAINING: "I came to Todd in the spring of 2004, after a very so-so year. I needed to elevate my production on the field. After years of training in the same 'Eastern European' style of Olympic lifting, my body and mind were looking for a fresh start. All the years of neglecting my core, feet, ankles—my foundation as a linebacker—left me unsteady and weak."

WHEN HE REALIZED IMPACT MADE A DIFFERENCE: "It wasn't a moment, but a span of time from that first off-season to the end of my first regular season. It was the best I'd felt in years. Todd really helped my body get primed for all the unpredictable body movements that take place in football. I have enjoyed much more success on the field since the start of my training, and I owe a lot of it to Todd."

HIS TRAINING SECRET: "Nutrition. It's impossible to set goals for your workout programs and have all these expectations of how you want your body and mind to be at the end when you don't give yourself the proper nutritional foundation. You have to put the right foods in your body before each workout to give your muscles something to feed on during the workout; and, more importantly, give it the right building blocks for recovery after. I'd ask people to listen to their bodies more before and after they eat, and get a feel for what foods make them feel good and which ones make them feel bad. You'll notice that the better foods always make you feel better."

What About Dairy?

Hey, I love dairy, but many Americans struggle to break down the sugar in milk (lactose), which causes digestive problems. This doesn't mean you need to avoid all dairy products, or the healthy nutrients they provide. Milk, cheese, yogurt, and cottage cheese are great options that provide calcium and a convenient boost of protein. Incorporate these foods into your nutrition plan, but practice moderation—one to three servings of dairy per day. If dairy causes you digestive discomfort, look for lactose-free versions or try alternatives like almond milk.

Two Meals for the Price of One

Restaurant visits can destroy your IMPACT nutrition program. It's no longer just McDonald's—every restaurant serves "supersize" meals without you asking for them. It has become almost impossible to separate healthy from unhealthy options. Portion size, calorie count, and sodium content are off the charts. Here's a tip: Ask your waiter or waitress to put half of your order in a doggie bag before you're even served. It's the easiest way to guarantee a healthier dining experience, and you end up with two meals for the price of one.

1 Get Your Motor Started: Eat Breakfast!

Breakfast is a meal important enough to merit its own section in this book. Think about this for a minute: The people in this world who live the longest never skip breakfast. Now . . . consider how often you skip the first meal of the day. I know it's more often than you'll like to admit. And researchers at the University of Massachusetts Medical School found that those who didn't regularly eat breakfast were 450 percent more likely to be obese than those who started their day off with a meal. That alone should be enough to convince you to make 10 extra minutes for breakfast. But there's more.

When you wake up in the morning, your body is in a fasting state in which it hasn't taken in nutrients for approximately 7 to 9 hours. Put that in perspective: Imagine not eating from 9:00 a.m. until 5:00 p.m. You'd be pretty hungry, wouldn't you? And because you want fuel in your tank at all times, the morning is the most important time of day to supercharge your engine.

The perfect breakfast isn't as complicated as it sounds. Scrambled eggs, some spinach and peppers, and a glass of almond milk is a great example. Eggs are a quality source of protein, and a study in the *Journal of Obesity* found that eating eggs in the morning leads to 65 percent more weight loss and an increase in energy.

TD's personal quick-fix pick: If I have an early start to the day, I love waking up to a

---

IMPACT tip /// Each morning, eat a combination of protein and carbohydrates, and even a little fat, which means a bagel and coffee won't cut it. Neither will a box of cereal that looks like it belongs in a Saturday morning cartoon. Cereal isn't off-limits, but make sure you avoid options that contain more than 10 grams of sugar per serving or have a long list of unpronounceable ingredients and zero fiber. When done right, a good breakfast speeds weight loss, helps you build lean muscle, and starts your day off right.

delicious protein shake that gets my day started right. Try the "Rise and Shine" Breakfast Shake, found on page 84. If you don't want a shake, try one of my all-time MVP breakfasts:

◗ Bowl of oatmeal (1 cup), raisins, blueberries, bananas, and slivered almonds with a pinch of cinnamon and a scoop of whey protein powder, or an omelet (three eggs) with spinach, salsa, avocado, and two slices of Ezekiel bread. Include a glass of orange juice (not concentrate) mixed with Green Vibrance greens drink.

2 Slow Down!

We're a gluttonous society. Big cars, big houses, and big appetites. We're always in a hurry. And we're also addicted to instant gratification. When you apply that to food, you have too many people shoveling in too much food way too fast. It takes the brain 20 minutes to process how much you're eating, so when you make your food vanish as fast as Sid, my golden retriever, your brain doesn't have time to cut you off, and you consume far more food than you need.

Why does this happen? Because you're hungry! If you never felt hungry, then the binges would stop. The best way to fix this? Eat more frequently and consume small amounts each time. Ideally, you'll eat five or six times a day—three small meals and two or three snacks. The grazing approach

Breakfasts on the Go

Grab any one of these nutritious options first thing in the morning if you're short on time. Each can be made in less than 5 minutes.

1 Whole wheat English muffin, 2 tablespoons of almond butter, and a handful of blueberries

2 Two slices of Ezekiel bread or 100 percent whole wheat bread, 1 tablespoon of jam, an orange, and two hard-boiled eggs

3 1 cup of oatmeal (no added sugar) mixed with raisins, walnuts, and 1 scoop of whey protein powder

What Is It?
EZEKIEL BREAD

I love Ezekiel bread. It's a nutrient-dense bread made from wheat, barley, lentils, and other natural ingredients that is higher in protein and fiber than most other breads. You'll find it listed throughout the IMPACT nutrition plan, and it can be found in most health-food outlets.

IMPACT tip /// Become a smarter shopper. Choose markets that offer fresh options, such as Trader Joe's, Whole Foods, Fresh Market, Wegmans, or, best of all, your local farmer's market. (Bonus tip: Make friends with a local butcher—you'll get higher-quality cuts of meat, and he'll direct you to what's really good that week.) As a rule of thumb, spend less time in the aisles and more time working the perimeter. If it's perishable, eat it. If you can't pronounce the ingredients, avoid it. The smarter you shop, the better you'll eat.

will prevent the binges. And remember: Eat slowly. Savor it! Enjoy the moment! When you do this right, you'll always be satisfied, you'll never overeat, and you'll provide your body with the nutrients it needs to remain energetic all day.

There's another big reason to eat smaller, more frequent meals: blood sugar and insulin spikes that occur after you eat. Insulin is a hormone that has both fat-storing and muscle-building properties. When you eat, especially carbohydrates and sugar, your blood glucose level rises quickly. This stimulates the release of insulin, which is a powerful hormone that tells your body to store fat. The more foods you eat that cause your blood glucose to increase, the higher your insulin levels increase, and your body stays in fat-gaining mode for a longer period of time. (Remember metabolic syndrome?)

But insulin isn't all bad. If you eat at the right times and learn how to prevent dramatic increases and drops in blood glucose, you can actually lose weight and put on muscle! How? By sticking with the eating plan in this chapter. You'll keep your body constantly fueled with nutrient-dense foods that don't cause blood sugar and insulin spikes, which means that throughout the day your metabolic engine will run at a steady, healthy level—not in a constant series of peaks and valleys that stress your liver and pancreas. This also means you'll curb sudden food cravings, eat less overall, and lose weight faster.

5 POWER HERBS AND SPICES

By Christopher R. Mohr, PhD, RD

1 TURMERIC This is the ultimate anti-inflammatory spice. Add it to rice, veggie dishes, or even scrambled eggs!

2 CINNAMON Another powerful spice. Just ½ teaspoon per day has been shown to lower LDL ("bad") cholesterol and triglycerides, and may lower blood sugar in those with diabetes. It's also a powerful antioxidant. Sprinkle some on oatmeal, cottage cheese, or yogurt, or try it in your postworkout smoothie.

3 OREGANO Just 1 teaspoon of this potent herb has as many antioxidants as ½ cup of chopped asparagus! Add it to Italian dishes, or sprinkle some on salads or soups.

4 GINGER This favorite holiday spice has been shown to have some strong anti-inflammatory properties, which is great for the workout fanatic and weekend warrior. Mix some in stir-fries and soups, and use it anytime you want to add a little Asian flare to your dishes.

5 RED PEPPER FLAKES (or cayenne pepper, which is the powdered version of the same) While some data suggest that an ingredient in red pepper flakes, capsaicin, may have fat-burning properties, other studies point to the powerful antioxidants in this spice. Try adding a pinch to sauces or chili when you want a little extra kick.

IMPACT tip /// Your days are busy, which makes it easy to forget to have frequent meals. But that's the first step that leads to overeating. Set your watch to go off as a reminder, and remember these two numbers:

3 The ideal number of waking hours between one IMPACT meal or snack and the next

5 The maximum number of waking hours to go without eating an IMPACT meal or snack

3 Fuel Up before Training

A high-quality workout doesn't begin with your dynamic warmup, activation exercises, or even tying your shoes. The process starts with your preworkout meal. This is the first step to getting your body right so it can perform at optimal levels. If you're training to become at least 1 percent better each time, you need to supply your body with the right foods.

Back when I was growing up in New Jersey, there was lots of talk about "fat-burning zones." People would wake up early, not eat anything, and then run for miles. Pushing your body like this on an empty tank is a recipe for disaster. The same holds true before the IMPACT workouts. When you eat before your workout, those calories won't be stored as fat. That's energy you'll use to run, jump, throw, and lift better than ever before. Eat an IMPACT snack or light meal approximately 1 to 2 hours before your IMPACT workout and you will be ready to set your body's metabolism on fire.

4 Refuel after Training

Your body isn't built in the gym. You actually break muscle down during a workout. Afterward, muscles become spongelike and want to soak up nutrients so they can rebuild themselves stronger and leaner while you rest. Plus, even when you are finished with your IMPACT workouts, your metabolism and hormones will be revved for hours. To aid this process, it's critical to refuel right after a workout. I recommend eating something within 30 minutes of training and certainly no longer than 1 hour afterward. The best part: During this window of "eating opportunity," your fat-storing enzymes take a short vacation, meaning you're primed to eat and not worry about adding a few inches to your waist—though this is not a ticket to binge. Remember, nutrition is about giving your body what it needs, not starving it, and not overfeeding it.

5 Go Wild!

Technological advancements provide us with a lot of great food options and better food safety. But our ancestors had the right idea: Fresh food is better. I've never seen an obese person who got fat because they ate too much fruit, salad, and fish. Eat fresh and wild and you will be eating better! In other words, if it comes from the ground, it's probably healthy. If it's from above ground, the fewer legs it has, the better. So lean toward fish before chicken, and chicken before beef. Still a little unsure? If your food has a longer shelf life than most of your relationships, put it down and find a new option.

Next to vegetables and fruit, organic meats and fresh wild fish are the best foundations for

(continued on page 86)

IMPACT tip /// About 1 to 2 hours before my workout, I like to snack on one of the following options:

/ **Greek yogurt and almonds**

/ **Fruit and nuts**

/ **Larabar or Optimal Nutrition 91 Bars** (Chewy chocolate chip is my favorite. Find them at www.optimalnutritioninc.com.)

/ **Pecans and a pear**

10 TASTY PROTEIN SHAKE RECIPES

Use any of these recipes to start your day, fuel up before a workout, or replenish your muscles after you've finished training. In any of the shakes, feel free to add 1 tablespoon of ground flaxseed and go with extra ice or no ice.

||||||||||||||||||||||||||||||||||||||||||||||||||||||||||||||||||

TD Quickie

6 ounces water, juice, or almond milk

1 scoop egg white powder or whey protein isolate

6 ice cubes

Shake, stir, or blend, and enjoy!

TD's Fat Burner

12 ounces water or unsweetened almond milk

2 scoops egg white powder or whey protein isolate

8 strawberries

1 tablespoon raw almond butter or ground flaxseed

6 ice cubes

Mix in a blender for 30 seconds.

TD's Preworkout Shake

8–12 ounces water

2 scoops egg white powder or whey protein isolate

1 banana

6 ice cubes

Mix in a blender for 30 seconds.

TD's Daddy Shake (My kids love it!)

12 ounces fresh orange juice

2 scoops egg white powder or whey protein isolate

1 banana

2 tablespoons almond butter or natural peanut butter

6 ice cubes

Shake, stir, or blend.

TD's Tropical Delight Shake

12 ounces water or orange juice

1 scoop whey protein isolate

¼ cup each of as many fruits as you can find in the fridge

1 banana

6 ice cubes

Mix in a blender for 30 seconds.

TD's Post–Game/ Practice/Workout Recovery Shake

12 ounces water

2 scoops whey protein isolate

Before your event or workout, fill an empty water bottle with protein powder. After your event, add water and shake vigorously for 30 seconds.

TD's "Rise and Shine" Breakfast Shake

12–16 ounces fresh squeezed orange juice

2 scoops egg white powder or vanilla whey protein powder

1 banana

¼ cup Greek yogurt

2 teaspoons organic vanilla extract

1 tablespoon ground flaxseed (optional)

1 tablespoon lecithin (optional)

Blend together for 30 seconds.

Dr. Chris Mohr's Blueberry Blast

1 cup unsweetened vanilla almond milk

1 frozen banana (peel before freezing)

½ cup blueberries

1 scoop unflavored or vanilla protein powder

Mix in a blender for 30 seconds.

Tropical Breeze

1 cup unsweetened vanilla almond milk

1 cup frozen pineapple

1 teaspoon shredded coconut or coconut milk

½ cup frozen blueberries

1 scoop unflavored or vanilla protein powder

Mix in a blender for 30 seconds.

Dr. Chris Mohr's Chocolate Chip "Ice Cream"

1 cup unsweetened chocolate almond milk

1 tablespoon natural almond or peanut butter

1 frozen banana (peel before freezing)

1 tablespoon cacao nibs

1 cup raw spinach

1 scoop chocolate protein powder

Dash of red pepper flakes (optional)

Mix in a blender for 30 seconds.

IMPACT tip /// Within 30 to 60 minutes after you train, have either a recovery shake or a meal. If you have a shake, give it a little "and then some" and add 5 to 10 grams of glutamine, an amino acid that helps in muscle building and recovery. Here are some other terrific post-workout options: / **Sweet potato and a protein shake** / **Ezekiel bread with chicken or canned tuna and avocado**

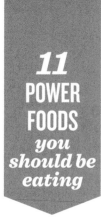

11 POWER FOODS *you should be eating*

BY CHRISTOPHER R. MOHR, PHD, RD

1 Sardines

These tiny fish are superhigh in omega-3 fats and have virtually no mercury, unlike many other fish. They're also a great source of calcium and vitamin D. They're sold year-round in cans. Add them to salads, mix them in pasta sauce, or use them in place of tuna.

2 Swiss chard

This dark green, leafy veggie is loaded with nutrients called carotenoids, which help protect your eyes. Sauté some chard with garlic and a bit of olive oil, and then add a pinch of salt and pepper.

3 Red cabbage

This cruciferous vegetable is packed with antioxidant polyphenols—particularly anthocyanins—which give red cabbage its color and may help protect your brain from Alzheimer's disease. Red cabbage also has up to eight times the vitamin C of white cabbage. Add shredded cabbage to wraps and salads, or Google "mayo-free coleslaw recipes" and give one a try!

4 Quinoa

(pronounced keen-wah) This ancient grain boasts one of the highest protein contents of any grain. It's also high in fiber and filled with more minerals than most grains have. It's great as a breakfast cereal, mixed with some dried fruit and nuts, or as a substitute for rice in recipes.

5 Broccoli

This vegetable is particularly high in a nutrient called sulforaphane, which has cancer-fighting properties. Mix broccoli into omelets, salads, stir-fries, and pasta sauce.

6 Black beans

Outside of fruits and vegetables, beans are one of the best forms of carbohydrates you can eat. They're loaded with fiber and protein, two reasons black beans help keep you full. A study in the *Journal of Agriculture and Food Chemistry* even showed that they have antioxidant levels comparable to those of cranberries and grapes! Add black beans to salads, wraps, and soups.

7 Garlic

Not only potent in your breath, garlic is also a potent antioxidant that may have antibacterial properties and reduce cholesterol, and research shows it boosts your immunity. Slice, chop, or mince garlic at least 10 minutes before using it to receive the most benefit. Add it to soups, sauces, eggs, or sautéed veggies.

8 Pistachios

In its shell, the pistachio is often referred to as "the skinny nut." That's because taking the time to break pistachios open limits how quickly they can be eaten. Combined with their high fiber and protein content, these nuts are hard to beat for nutrient value.

9 Blueberries

These tiny nutrient powerhouses should be a regular part of your diet. Blueberries are linked to improved mental functioning, a benefit that can be attributed to anthocyanins—compounds that give the fruit its dark color. Pick up a bag of frozen berries and add them to smoothies or yogurt.

10 Fat-free Greek yogurt

This product is fairly new to the scene—at least in terms of popularity. Greek yogurt is strained, but that means it has double the protein and half the sugar! It has a much thicker consistency than regular yogurt but works really well in smoothies, and even as a base ingredient in place of mayonnaise for egg or chicken salad.

11 Tea

(green, black, or white): Several cups each day may keep the doctor away! Research has shown that drinking tea may boost immunity, reduce the risk of heart disease, and even improve mental function. Your best bet: Brew your own. The bottled options typically have so much sugar that the products barely qualify as tea.

your main meals. While organic might cost a little more, it's devoid of pesticides, herbicides, fungicides, and other toxic compounds that you don't want. And farm-raised fish contains higher levels of mercury and bacteria than wild fish does. Remember, in this program you're striving for a high-performance body. If you settle for low-quality fuel, you'll receive low-quality energy.

6 Remember That Supplements Are Just That—Supplements!

A lot of people are looking for a magic pill to change their bodies. They want results faster than those results can realistically occur. Sorry, folks, the world doesn't work that way. This program is designed to maximize your body's potential, and you'll do that through cutting-edge training and world-class effort. Sometimes the supplement industry would have you believe that what it sells are magic pills, but trust me, they aren't. However, the right ones can be incredibly beneficial. Supplements help fill any unforeseen gaps in your nutrition, and they allow your body to function at its highest level.

Supplements get a bad rap because they're not regulated by the Food and Drug Administration. That just means you need to be smart about what you purchase. The label on any supplement can be scary reading. There are lots of ingredients and enough warnings that you feel you need a lawyer to translate them. Don't worry: I'll show you the supplements that can help you the most, the ones that science has shown to be beneficial—and the supplements that I trust and take myself.

Just remember, a supplement is just a supplement, and not a replacement for food. No magic pills, my friend.

YOUR DAILY IMPACT SUPPLEMENTS

Your supplement needs can easily be grouped into two categories: those that help your overall health, wellness, and vitality, and those that target your recovery, regeneration, and joint health. Use this guide to choose what's best for you.

HEALTH, WELLNESS, AND VITALITY SUPPLEMENTS

Multivitamin

The all-in-one supplement will guarantee that you're receiving all your essential nutrients, including a healthy dose of antioxidants. If you're a man, watch out for iron. Unless you're deficient, adult men do not need to supplement iron in their diets. Women, you want just the opposite. Pick a product that supplies iron. I like liquid multivitamins for maximum absorption, and I make sure I consume it once a day.

TD'S PERSONAL PICK: First Choice liquid multivitamin

Greens drink

A greens drink is a great, effective way to start your day and receive a full range of antioxidants, vitamins, minerals, polyphenols, and probiotics. Probiotics (meaning "to promote life") are located in your intestinal tract and help reduce cholesterol, blood pressure, and inflammation, and improve your immune functioning. A good greens drink also supports your internal organs and helps keep you energized and healthy. Look for brands processed with protection from UV light, heat, and moisture, which maintains the nutrient content.

TD'S PERSONAL PICK: Green Vibrance by Vibrant Health

Vitamin B Complex

If food is your fuel, then a vitamin B complex is high-grade oil helping your engine run better. B vitamins assist with almost every process and system in your body, including healthy digestion; a strong nervous system; good hair, skin, and nails; and, maybe most important, energy production. That's because vitamin B helps convert carbohydrates into glucose, which your body then converts into energy. (You might know this as your metabolism.) If you drink coffee or alcohol, your need for vitamin B increases.

TD'S PERSONAL PICK: Look for the following vitamins in any complex: B1 (thiamine), B2 (riboflavin), B3 (niacin), B5 (pantothenic acid), B6 (pyridoxine), B9, B12, and biotin, choline, folic acid, and inositol.

Ground Flaxseed

These little seeds help reduce your risk of heart disease, cancer, stroke, and diabetes. Just make sure they're ground—buy it that way or use a coffee grinder or blender. Sprinkle ground flaxseed on your salads, into protein shakes, or on yogurt to fortify your meals with extra vitamins, minerals, healthy fats, and fiber. Take in 2 to 4 tablespoons daily.

TD'S PERSONAL PICK: Barlean's 100% Organic Forti-Flax

Vitamin D

Scientists have determined that vitamin D plays a vital role in building strong bones, fighting cancer, protecting your body against infection, and helping bust your gut and aiding in fat loss. Don't assume that you're getting enough vitamin D from your diet. Research indicates that 60 percent of Americans are deficient. Visit your doctor and check whether your levels are normal. A good result is between 50 and 80 nanograms per milliliter.

TD'S PERSONAL PICK: Look for a product with at least 1,000 international units. (Also, Nordic Naturals Ultimate Omega with D is vitamin D–enhanced omega-3 fish oil, which kills two birds with one stone. See "Omega-3's.")

Green Tea Extract

Green tea extract offers one of the best sources of antioxidants, which are important to your health because they fight off dangerous free radicals, the primary cause of aging in your body. In addition, green tea extract revs up your metabolism, boosts cardiovascular health, offers sustained energy, and even improves skin quality. Just keep an eye on the label. Avoid products that include caffeine, sugar, artificial sweeteners, preservatives, alcohol, gluten, or calories.

TD'S PERSONAL PICK: Pure Inventions Green Tea Extract—peach flavor!

RECOVERY, REGENERATION, AND JOINT HEALTH SUPPLEMENTS

Protein Powders

There's no shortage of protein options on the shelves of your local health food store. Whey protein isolate (WPI) is the highest grade of whey protein currently available, and it's quickly and easily digested into your muscles. WPI is also a great source of branched chain amino acids (BCAAs), which are the building blocks of protein synthesis, or your ability to build muscle. The next-best thing to WPI is egg protein. The biggest difference between the two is that egg is absorbed into your body at a slower rate. This makes it perfect for a meal replacement option, while WPI is ideal for before or after your workout. I recommend one to two protein shakes per day, typically before and/or after your workout.

TD'S PERSONAL PICK: EAS Whey Protein Isolate, Jay Robb Whey Protein Powder Isolate, or Jay Robb Egg White Protein Powder

Glutamine

If you're looking for one supplement to help with recovery from your IMPACT workouts, look no further. Glutamine is the most common amino acid found in your muscles, and during intense training (like the type you'll be doing), glutamine levels are depleted, which reduces your strength, stamina, and recovery. Supplementing with glutamine will not only increase your lean muscle tissue, but can also boost growth hormone levels and aid your immune system. I recommend consuming 10 grams per day, splitting it between after your workout and before bed.

TD'S PERSONAL PICK: EAS Glutamine

Joint Support

Here's the closest thing we have to dipping your joints in the fountain of youth. Joint products that combine glucosamine, chondroitin, and MSM may help stimulate the production of healthy cartilage and improve the integrity of connective soft tissue. The bottom line: Your joints and connective tissues—including fascia, as well as your tendons and ligaments—will feel less pain when you take these supplements. Look for products that consist of 1.5 grams of glucosamine, 1.2 grams of chondroitin, and between 300 and 900 milligrams of MSM.

TD'S PERSONAL PICK: Advocare Joint ProMotion or GNC TriFlex

Fish oils

Eating fish, nuts, and seeds isn't the only way to provide healthy fats to your body. These options supply endless health benefits, including great support for your joints. Choose one of the following if you choose to supplement healthy oils.

OMEGA-3'S: Omega-3 fatty acids are involved in the metabolism of every cell in your body. They act as metabolic spark plugs that help spur fat loss, reduce heart disease and stroke, fight inflammation, and offer brain-boosting benefits. Look for the terms EPA and DHA on the label—these are both omega-3 fats. The American Heart Association recommends 4 grams total of EPA and DHA per day, depending on your health risk. Be sure to check with your doctor if you take medications such as Coumadin or aspirin, as fish oils can thin your blood.

TD'S PERSONAL PICK: Nordic Naturals fish oils. (Also, as I mentioned earlier, Nordic Naturals Ultimate Omega with D includes a dose of vitamin D, which takes care of two supplements in one.)

Tip: If your breath smells like fish or you are burping it up, consider a different brand or look for enteric-coated fish oils.

COD LIVER OIL: This is a terrific alternative to omega-3 fish oil supplements. This healthy fat provides a spectrum of benefits, including high levels of omega-3 fatty acids and vitamins A and D, and it helps fight joint pain and arthritis. When taken by pregnant women, cod liver oil helps the brain development and overall health of newborn babies.

TD'S PERSONAL PICK: Carlson's Norwegian Cod Liver Oil

7 Water Your Body

When I played football at The College of William & Mary, we had an odd ritual during summer two-a-day workouts. Before each practice, the trainers would examine the color of our urine as we stood at the urinal. If it was too yellow (like apple juice), we'd have to sit out practice due to dehydration. If it looked like pale lemonade, we were good to go. While the tradition was always a bit weird, our trainers knew what they were doing. A dehydrated body is programmed for failure.

Our bodies are about 70 percent water, meaning we need to hydrate as often as possible. In other words, drink more water! How much? I like to say half of your body weight in fluid ounces daily. So if you're a 180-pound man, you should consume at least 90 ounces (or about 11 cups) of water each day. If you're drinking caffeinated drinks, fruit juices, or alcohol, you'll need even more. Regardless, most of us live in a dehydrated state and don't even realize it. Remember, if your urine isn't clear or a pale yellow like lemonade, you're not drinking enough water.

Water is also an ally of muscle growth, and your secret weapon against hunger. Water improves exercise performance, lubricates your joints, increases disk cushioning in your spine, and even keeps your skin healthy and slows the aging process. But, maybe best of all, drinking more water can help you

MAKE CAFFEINE WORK FOR YOU

My days often start early. I'm an energetic guy, but I also enjoy an occasional caffeine boost. In fact, it has been shown that caffeine increases your performance and energy in the gym and can help you achieve a world-class workout. One cup of coffee won't kill you, but when we rely on too much caffeine, we stop receiving benefits and start building dependencies. Keep your caffeine consumption to 150 to 200 milligrams total per day (that's 1 to 2 cups of coffee or 3 to 4 cups of black tea). And avoid all the cream, sugar, whipped cream, and other junk that people often add to it, as that will pack on excess calories and reap you no nutritional benefits. Example: A Starbucks Venti White Chocolate Mocha has 580 calories (a Grande has 470 calories), and both have 150 milligrams of caffeine.

IMPACT tip /// Water doesn't have to be boring. Use these suggestions to spike your drink, improve its taste, and add additional health benefits.

/ After a workout, opt for coconut water. It is low in calories and sugar, and is high in electrolytes.

/ Mix in green tea extract to add numerous health benefits (see Your Daily IMPACT Supplements) and sustained energy.

/ Add slices of lemons to your water. Lemon helps alkalize water and acts as a natural detoxifier. Most foods are acidic, and lemon (an alkaline) helps balance your digestive system.

keep your weight down. Sometimes when you feel hungry, it's actually thirst. When you drink more water, your belly's full, you're less likely to overeat, and your body will function at a higher level.

8 Keep a Nutrition Journal

Research indicates that we lie to ourselves: We overestimate how much we exercise and underestimate how much we eat. You can stop that now if you keep track of everything you consume, even water. How has your nutrition improved? What new foods have you tried and loved? How have your energy levels improved? What new strategies have you found to push past cravings? What new healthy eating habit do you want to try this week? A nutrition journal can be a crucial improvement to your life. You'll be more in control of what you eat and how you think about eating. This can be one serious high-performance habit. Try it for a week and see what it reveals.

9 Follow the 90-10 Rule

This program is all about putting you in control of your life, which includes what you eat. Throughout this book, I've been encouraging you to be your best. 10 in–10 out. It's a formula built for success, and one that teaches you to expect great things from your life. But if there's one exception to the rule, it's in nutrition. If you strive to be perfect with everything you eat, you'll fail. That's what we want to avoid. People will eat healthy during the week, and when the weekend hits, they have a Saturday cheat day that turns into a 2-day junk-food bender.

I believe in the 90-10 rule. If 90 percent of the time you eat the right foods, you're going to look world class, feel great, and achieve your goals. It's that simple. For the other 10 percent, allow yourself to sample foods that you love, and don't confine yourself to perfection. Just don't let it spin out of control. It'll keep your nutrition in line and you in control of your success.

10 Experiment with the IMPACT Menu

When you think about the IMPACT menu, imagine foods that offer your body everything it could ever want or need: fulfilling flavor-filled meals that are diverse and satisfying, and ensure that you will look good and function even better. Now stop imagining and start eating! IMPACT nutrition is a no-stress approach that allows you to experiment and enjoy a variety of foods across the dietary spectrum— including carbs, protien, and fats.

I promise, you've never eaten better. I'm not talking about microwave vegetables and frozen chicken breasts. Get away from take-out and

---

IMPACT tip /// If you decide to save your entire 10 percent for 1 day, you're kidding yourself. You're adding stress and negativity to a 9-day stretch of perfect eating, and then setting yourself up for 1 day of salt, sugar, and empty calories. It's too easy to overindulge, so remind yourself of your goals, revel in the foods you can eat all the time, allow yourself the occasional indulgence, and you'll stay within the proven success of the 90-10 rule.

fast-food and get to know your kitchen a little bit better (1 percent every day). You can always use a cookbook and learn how to grill meat, fish, veggies, and even fruit. After all, when your entire dinner has only four or five ingredients, how hard could it be?

I will not dictate what you eat. I realize that each of us has unique tastes and preferences, so if you don't like something shown here, substitute your favorite. My goal is to get your mouth watering with a menu of simply prepared, fresh ingredients—because IMPACT nutrition will move you one step closer to improving your energy and wellness. Ready to eat?

The next step is yours to take.

I KNOW THAT FOOD ACCOUNTS for only one chapter in this book, but I cannot stress this enough: How you eat will help determine your ultimate success with the IMPACT program. Again, there are no shortcuts. Food is fuel, and fuel determines how your engine runs. That's it. That's the key for you. And look at what an amazing array of foods you have at your fingertips! My mouth waters every time I read this section, because we're not talking about bland, boring choices. We're talkin' savory, versatile, nutrient-dense, easy-to-prepare food that you don't have to worry about eating, because it's all good. Just eat, baby! Easy, right?

But nutrition is just one part of the IMPACT program that takes place outside the gym. In fact, another critical aspect of the program happens when you're not working out. Proper (or improper) rest, recovery, and regeneration will determine how your body rebuilds (or doesn't rebuild) itself between workouts. The next chapter will teach you all you need to know about respecting your body and the downtime it needs to remake itself into something greater, something 1 percent better than it was yesterday. You need this info, my friend. So let's get after it!

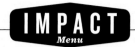

BREAKFAST

Include fruit with all breakfast suggestions.
Take a good liquid multivitamin
and B12 every morning.

Oatmeal with raisins, berries, nuts,
and 1 scoop of protein powder

Omelet with vegetable medley

Ezekiel bread with almond butter, apple butter,
or organic, all-natural peanut butter

Bagel and lox with capers, tomatoes, and onions

Yogurt or granola with fresh fruit and nuts

Protein shake made with fresh fruit or peanut butter

Whole grain cereal or muesli with fresh fruit and
choice of organic milk, almond milk, or rice milk

Multigrain pancakes or waffles
with almond butter and fresh fruit

2 or 3 hard-boiled eggs with 1 slice
of whole wheat bread, jam, and grapefruit

Toasted whole wheat English muffin with
2 tablespoons of almond butter, and blueberries

Scrambled eggs, spinach, onion, and bell pepper
with 1 slice of cheese in a whole wheat flour tortilla

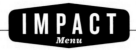

LUNCH AND DINNER

Include salad and greens with each meal.
For salad dressing, use olive oil and lemon, or flaxseed oil.
Sauté vegetables in coconut oil, with garlic and onion.
Use fresh herbs and lemon zest for extra flavor.

Salad greens tossed with olive oil and lemon,
served with grilled chicken or fish

Grilled or roasted wild salmon
brushed with olive oil, served with chickpeas,
mixed greens, and balsamic vinaigrette

Sliced grilled chicken breast
with minced ginger, red onion, bell pepper, and
chili sauce, served on a bed of brown rice

Chunk albacore tuna with avocado
on whole grain bread or wrap

Sliced roast turkey or chicken breast with avocado
and arugula on whole grain bread or wrap

Whole wheat linguine or angel-hair pasta,
marinara sauce, and vegetable medley, served with
grilled shrimp or chicken

Baked halibut fillet brushed
with Dijon mustard and olive oil, topped with red
onion and bell pepper, on a bed of quinoa

Grilled tuna steak with fresh lemon,
sautéed or steamed vegetable medley, and couscous

Grilled or poached fish or chicken with grilled, thick-
sliced sweet potato and choice of green vegetable

Chicken and vegetable stir-fry, sliced scallion,
and carrots with brown rice

Turkey or chicken burger, lettuce, tomato,
and red onion on optional whole wheat bun

Thin-sliced lean beef tenderloin on a bed of spring
greens with cherry tomatoes, shaved Parmesan, olive
oil, and a drizzle of lemon juice

Sliced grilled or roasted pork tenderloin,
crumbled feta cheese, bell pepper, and mixed greens
with a drizzle of balsamic vinaigrette

Homemade bean soup

White bean chili (vegetarian, turkey, or chicken)

Grilled flank steak, corn on the cob,
mixed greens, and balsamic vinaigrette

Whole wheat spaghetti with marinara sauce,
turkey meatballs, and Swiss chard

Sliced roast turkey breast with hummus
and butter lettuce or sprouts on 2 slices of toasted
whole wheat bread

Sautéed chicken breast
with steamed spinach and bok choy

Roasted wild salmon fillet
on a bed of fresh arugula with whole wheat orzo,
shaved Parmesan cheese, and fresh lemon juice

Grilled pork tenderloin, cucumber slices with Greek
yogurt, and grilled peach halves with a honey drizzle

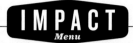

IMPACT
Menu

S N A C K S

Men: *Aim for approximately 250 to 400 calories per snack.*
Women: *Aim for approximately 150 to 300 calories per snack.*

~

Piece of fruit: apple, banana, orange, or pear

~

Protein shake

~

Protein bar (Shoot for bars that are low in sugar and have a short ingredient list.)

~

Cashews, pecans, pistachios, or walnuts (1 handful)

~

Fresh berries

~

Carrots and hummus

~

Almond butter and apple

~

Yogurt and nuts

~

Hard-boiled egg

~

Roast beef, celery, and whole wheat crackers

9
SLEEP, RECOVERY, AND REGENERATION

 "Since you were born, what has your body done for you? Since you were born, what have you done for your body?"

—ZEN PROVERB

Is life a marathon or a sprint?

I was asked the same thing years ago by one of my mentors, Wayne Cotton. I promptly answered, "Life's a marathon. You keep running and running, and whoever goes the longest wins." Wayne looked at me, chuckled, and told me something that changed my life.

"No, Todd. Life is a series of sprints. You sprint, sprint, sprint, and then rest and recover. That way, you're always exerting maximum effort for the best results, but you rest so you don't burn out. If you just keep sprinting, you're going to die."

That moment helped me understand why I felt fatigued even when I was exercising and eating right. I needed to relax more. We sprint and seldom stop. We're like hamsters on a wheel, going round and round, and if we keep pushing ourselves all the time, eventually we're going to break down. Guaranteed. If you want to be filled with energy, decrease your stress, and change the way you live, then you need to change what you've been doing. You need to sleep, take time to recover, and go the extra mile to help your body regenerate and cope with the hundreds of daily stressors in your life. Otherwise, you're begging to hit a wall, be run over by life, and end up another statistic, because you choose not to change.

If you looked at your day-to-day existence, what would you see? For most people, it's chaos. You live in a stressful world where you're juggling work, kids, relationships, financial responsibilities, and social obligations. And after all that, you still need to factor in exercise and rest—the foundations of a world-class existence. And yet those are usually the first things you neglect. We disregard ourselves, and watch as our health and happiness fall short of our hopes and expectations.

I realize you might be thinking, "Todd, you want me to slow down? I don't have time to slow down. There's too much to do. I'm stuck." Hey, I understand that. I genuinely do. I have a wife and three young kids. I run my facility, Fitness Quest 10, with 35 teammates, direct the Under Armour Performance Training Council, have numerous speaking engagements around the country, and mentor many fitness entrepreneurs. Through all that, I still have to be the best husband, father, trainer, mentor, and boss I can be. And even as a gym owner, it's just as hard for me to sneak in a workout. But I'll share a secret with you: You can't handle all your responsibilities without scheduled "me time." If it doesn't get scheduled, it doesn't get in. But nothing will change until you give yourself permission to slow down. Prioritize these strategies for recovery and regeneration, and help set your mind and body right.

By now, you have seen that I ask a lot out of my clients with their fitness. I truly believe that through physical conditioning, you can change your life.

DON'T WAIT, TAKE CONTROL

We live in a reactive world. We often wait until something happens, and then we react. This is why our health sometimes fails. We're so busy sprinting that we don't stop until our bodies shut down and force us to take notice of the damage we've done. Instead, take a proactive attitude and prevent stress from overwhelming your system. Focus on your body with exercise and prioritize your mind by scheduling downtime to ensure your well-being. We all want to go fast and accomplish more goals than there is time for in a day. But sometimes you have to go slow in order to go fast. By recharging your batteries and taking care of your health, you set a foundation that will have you feeling great and able to perform optimally!

But as hard as you condition, you must place just as much emphasis on your recovery. And while nutrition plays a vital role in this process, there are other aspects that are integral to complete regeneration and overall health. Sleep, massage, bodywork, and breath work are all essential parts of this program that will help your mind and body feel refreshed and rejuvenated.

What Is Recovery? /// Recovery refers to any techniques you use to relax and improve your body. Recovery strategies should be applied to both your mental and physical needs. Some great ones are sleep, massage, yoga, World-Class Eating, and vacation. When all else fails, just lean back in your chair and breathe.

Sleep

"Sleep restores and optimizes our metabolism, memory, focus, creativity, mental processing speed, emotional balance, musculoskeletal performance, and immune defenses. And that's just for starters. . . ." —Mindy Cetel, MD, FAASM

Sleep is more than a place where dreams come true. It's the foundation that helps you function at your highest level. After a good night of rest, you feel refreshed, reenergized, and ready to own the day. And yet rarely, if ever, do you prioritize sleep or think about how it influences every function in your body. Maybe you can run on adrenaline for a little while, but eventually the sleep deficit catches up with you. A lack of sleep is associated with poor metabolism, bad lipid profiles, higher blood pressure, adrenal fatigue, less muscle, and a greater likelihood of suffering from obesity. Need proof? People who sleep 4 hours or less per night are 70 percent more likely to be overweight! And those same sleep-deprived people are more likely to overeat. It's a vicious cycle that starts with not sleeping enough.

When you sleep, your body is in full recovery mode. Your brain refreshes itself so you can think and process information clearly, while your muscles rebuild so you can look and feel better. That's partially because sleep influences the hormones in your body. Uninterrupted sleep boosts growth hormone and testosterone, which help you recover quicker, feel better, have more energy, build more lean muscle tissue, and even age

FIND YOUR STRESS BAROMETER

We all have barometers to gauge our stress, if we listen. For me, it's my lower back. When my stress level is too high, my lower back stiffens and serves as a warning sign that if I don't slow down or spend enough time on my recovery strategies, my back may put me down for a few days. What warning signs does your body use to signal you? Headaches, upper-back and neck tension, lower-back pain. Is your body telling you something? If so, are you listening?

> ## "Take rest; a field that has rested gives a beautiful crop."
>
> — OVID

What Is Regeneration? /// In biology, regeneration refers to the regrowth of a cell after damage. While we can't guarantee you'll grow anything new (besides muscle!), regeneration occurs when you get enough rest to restore the quality of your soft tissue. That means your fascia, muscles, ligaments, and joints will feel like new again!

better. On the contrary, not sleeping enough increases cortisol, the stress hormone that makes your life miserable and turns your body into a storage room for fat. In other words: A well-rested body functions at its best.

So, what's the magic number? It varies with age, and there really isn't one correct answer. You have to find the amount that works for you. Six hours of sleep should be a minimum, and most research indicates that 7 to 8 hours is ideal. But, like almost anything else in life, too much sleep isn't good, either. The occasional 10-hour night is okay, but when it happens more frequently, it will ultimately shortchange your energy.

Instead of focusing just on hours, I also emphasize quality. Not all sleep is equal, and the better your sleep, the more energy you'll have to accomplish all your responsibilities, reach your goals, and still train hard. High-quality sleep also improves your mood and memory, and it boosts immunity so you're not as likely to be sick. I typically get about 7 hours of rest, all of which is high quality. That means I'm sleeping throughout the night with minimal disruptions, and I'm spending time in REM sleep, the restorative part of the sleep cycle, when dreams occur.

Unfortunately, too many of us suffer from sleep disruption, meaning we have trouble falling asleep or we wake up repeatedly during the night. Other

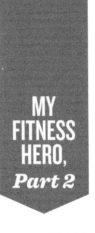

MY FITNESS HERO, *Part 2*

"AGE IS AN ISSUE OF MIND OVER MATTER. IF YOU DON'T MIND, IT DOESN'T MATTER."
—MARK TWAIN
Donna Dickinson's secret is nothing special. She follows the principles of the IMPACT program to a T and places special emphasis on recovery and regeneration. That means practicing an hour of yoga and breath work every morning. This keeps her fresh and allows her to enjoy working out 3 days per week and playing tennis 5 days per week. Her focus on taking care of her body is what allows her to have the vibrancy, energy, and strength that she does, even at the ripe young age of 70.

than emptying your bladder, you shouldn't be waking up. Either problem reduces your sleep quality and can disrupt your hormones. So even if you rest for 8 hours, if it's poor quality, you won't receive all the restorative and recovery benefits of a good night's sleep.

Upgrade Your Sleep /// If you're struggling to make it through the night, try one of these techniques, which can help you experience deep sleep and start living with more energy.

Have acupuncture treatments. • Avoid caffeine after noon. • Take magnesium (400 to 600 milligrams) 30 to 60 minutes before bedtime. • Visit your doctor and ask to have your adrenal glands and hormone levels checked. • Listen to a white-noise machine or relaxation CD. • Remove the TV from your bedroom. • Read. • Snack on walnuts a couple of hours before bed. • Purchase a new mattress. • Sleep in complete darkness. • Drink chamomile and lime blossom tea before sleeping. • Put lavender on your pillows.

Two common factors disrupt your sleep patterns: food and TV. Skip the late-night snacks and the midnight meals. Late-night eating can negatively affect your digestion. Every time you eat, it takes energy to fuel the digestive process and burn the food. (This is why you'll be eating frequently throughout the day on the IMPACT nutrition plan.) But when you eat before bed, the energy that should be spent on rejuvenating and reenergizing your cells and entire body is spent on digestion. You wake up tired, not refreshed, and generally confused about what you did wrong. Your body actually ends up spending too much time on digestion and not enough on recovery.

Another tip: Turn off the TV before you go to bed. If you fall asleep with the TV on, the electromagnetic waves and the light will force you to stay in a lighter sleep cycle and not get the restorative REM sleep you need to recover. The less time you spend in REM, the worse you'll feel the next morning. Or you might wake up to turn off the TV. This interruption disturbs your sleep pattern and decreases sleep quality. Ideally, turn off the TV 30 minutes before going to bed and listen to soft music or read a great book.

Recovery and Regeneration Techniques

I love showing up to work every day and seeing people get after it in my gym. And while my philosophy—and the one embraced by all my employees—is comprehensive and holistic, I still see too many folks on the edge of injury. Whether it's a lack of sleep, high stress, or too much time sitting at a desk, they can do a better job of maintaining their

IMPACT SECRETS *from the pros*

KELLEN WINSLOW
TIGHT END
TAMPA BAY BUCCANEERS

Todd Durkin client for 4 years

WHY HE NEEDS IMPACT TRAINING: "Todd knows how to adapt training to anyone's body and everyone's needs. Todd finds new ways to challenge my body, make me fast, keep me lean, and challenge my body while still keeping the workout focused on what I want. It's the reason I keep coming back. He makes working out more enjoyable no matter how difficult the program is."

WHEN HE REALIZED IMPACT MADE A DIFFERENCE : "I've never been a guy that enjoys lifting heavy weight all the time, but I'm in a sport where I need to be strong and explosive. Todd creates workouts that still make you stronger without putting too much stress on your joints. And he makes me faster and more explosive without having me feeling worn down. And for me, that's as important as anything."

HIS TRAINING SECRET: "Don't let weight training be your only type of fitness activity. You need to stay flexible with stretches and foam rolling, and you have to run, especially sprints. The faster you move, the better condition you're in. It's a great way to assess your fitness and know when you need to work a little harder."

When you're stressed, your breathing quickens, your breaths shorten, and your performance is affected. The key to calming yourself is managing your breathing, which helps you control your emotions and your health. A constricted oxygen supply limits your muscles' function and undercuts peak performance.

To improve oxygen flow, try nostril breathing for 10 minutes in the morning every few days, as a form of meditation. Lie flat on your back or sit upright and close your right nostril with your thumb alongside your nose as you inhale deeply through your left nostril. Take a deep breath. Then close your left nostril with your index finger, open your right nostril, and exhale. Inhale through your right nostril, then close it and exhale through the left. Repeat this pattern for 10 minutes, alternating deep inhales and exhales.

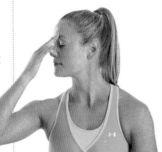

bodies. You see, most people fall into the misleading belief that doing strength work and cardio will keep you healthy. But when you don't emphasize recovery and regeneration, you end up falling short of your potential. I don't want that to be your story. Use these strategies to help your body function at its best.

Yoga and Pilates

If you remember when we described the Muscle Matrix back in Chapter 5, I mentioned that flexibility is one of the seven essential phases of the program. While stretching is one way to improve the flexibility of your muscles, yoga and Pilates offer another form of exercise that increases your flexibility, improves your structural alignment, and enhances your breathing.

We know that we're too tight. We feel it when we exercise, when we sit down, and when we try to lift anything off the floor. And yet we still ignore our pain. Your body is telling you (sometimes screaming at you) what's wrong, and yoga, Pilates, or any other concentrated stretching will help improve your flexibility and facilitate relaxation. If you are supertight, stretching for 10 minutes after your workout isn't enough. If you need to emphasize flexibility, prioritize it on a daily basis and feel free to do it multiple times a day.

And Then Some /// While I highly encourage you to start each morning with meditation or prayer, you can also do another session in the evening. Evening meditation eases your mind and helps you unwind after a long day. It also prepares your body for a more restful sleep. Consider doing nighttime meditation in addition to a morning session.

Another option is a gratitude journal. This exercise consists of writing down all the things you are thankful for in your life, such as the people, blessings, and opportunities. This simple practice can help shift your energy and improve your outlook.

Meditation and Breath Work

We breathe, on average, between 18,000 and 22,000 times per day. How often do you actually stop and pay attention to your breathing? Seldom to never, right? It's amazing, but the simple process of listening to your breath and focusing on it becomes a tremendous aid in feeling balanced, reducing stress, and controlling anxiety.

I am going to ask you to set aside 10 minutes every morning for meditation. Call it prayer time, quiet time, or whatever you want. I'm just asking that you take 10 minutes of "you time" to be quiet every morning. This helps you work on your inner self and sets the tone for your entire day. You can sit quietly, lie in corpse pose (called savasana in yoga), or even do "nostril breathing." (See "Catch Your Breath.")

Focus on deep belly breaths for 10 minutes. I often set a cooking timer for 10 minutes so that it will ring when my time is up. Quiet your mind and focus on your breath. And just breathe! If you do this, it will make a profound difference in your day. Try it for 10 days straight and see how you feel. Do it for 10 weeks and your life will be transformed.

Massage and Bodywork

Remember, my career in fitness and wellness began with massage and bodywork. It was Dub Leigh's work that altered my life and led me on a path to where I am today. I learned firsthand the multiple benefits of the power of touch, and how everyone, including people who are sedentary,

can experience numerous benefits from massage.

In 2002, I created Optimal Performance Bodywork (OPB), an eclectic mix of bodywork and exercise techniques that I used to heal my own back pain and avoid surgery. It is a form of soft-tissue bodywork that combines the best of myofascial release, Soft-Tissue Release, and Zen Bodytherapy. Of course, Zen Bodytherapy is Dub Leigh's work, which combines Rolfing, Feldenkrais, and energy work. Those techniques served as the core, in addition to countless other hands-on soft-tissue techniques that I learned and created along my journey.

The basic premise of OPB is that if your body is structurally aligned and in proper form, you can move freely and perform at optimum levels. (Visit www.FitnessQuest10.com for more information.) I spent 3 years exclusively teaching OPB around the country and spreading its benefits. It is now part of what I do and who I am. The ancient art of bodywork directly targets common problems and has restorative qualities that can help you relax.

Listen closely: Massage and bodywork is not a luxury. It's a necessity. As I told you in Chapter 4, "Secrets to a Pain-Free Body," everyday activities often worsen the quality of your fascia. Your body needs hands-on attention to function correctly, and by integrating massage and bodywork anywhere from once a week to once a month, you'll experience regenerative benefits for your mind and your body. The pliability and the quality of your fascia are improved by massage and bodywork. When you exercise or even sit for too long, adhesions build up in your connective tissues that restrict movement, comfort, and performance.

By addressing your fascia with human touch, you can remove muscle tension and stiffness, heal quicker from injuries, improve joint flexibility, and improve range of motion so you can move more efficiently and feel better.

But the forgotten benefit, and one that's important to improving how you feel, is that massage and bodywork creates awareness. I learned this from my sister Patti and from Dub Leigh. Oftentimes we suffer from a variety of aches and pains. Since the body is interconnected, your pain might be a symptom of a problem in another area of your body. It doesn't matter if your back hurts, your knees ache, or you have frequent headaches. Treating the symptom won't completely fix your issues. Massage and bodywork can treat the cause and make you feel better from head to toe. And that simple experience of feeling good, being relaxed, and experiencing no pain will show you what you should expect from your body.

WHAT TYPE OF MASSAGE *do you need?*

There are dozens of different types of massage. Some of the more common ones you'll see include Swedish (relaxation), deep tissue, sports, neuromuscular, myofascial release, Zen Bodytherapy, Optimal Performance Bodywork, Rolfing, hot stone, craniosacral, Reiki, lomilomi, Thai, Ashiatsu, Oriental Bar Therapy, Active Release Techniques (ART), and Muscle Activation Techniques (MAT), among many others. Check out www.amtamassage.org for descriptions of many of these different modalities to see which one might be best for you and to find a qualified therapist or bodyworker who might be right for you. Additionally, always select therapists who can tailor their routines to fit your goals. I'd recommend looking for someone with a National Certification Board for Therapeutic Massage & Bodywork (NCBTMB) certification.

Get Lost

Pull out your calendar and flip ahead 10 weeks. In that amount of time, you'll have finished the IMPACT transformation program. You'll be in better shape, healthier than ever, and feeling like a new person. Now look at your schedule and plan a vacation. Whether it's a long weekend or a tropical getaway, I want you to get lost. Reward yourself for your success with this program. Do something you love. Find adventure. Heck, come on down to San Diego and show your face at one of my workout classes. Don't make excuses or say you'll get around to creating adventure. Schedule it now. Make it happen, and it will serve as incentive and reward for your hard work and the effort you put into making changes. After all, this is about you creating an extraordinary life. And reward is one way to guarantee that your mind is right and your body is fresh.

The world isn't going to slow down anytime soon. Life is overwhelming at times, exhausting at others. But if you want to keep sprinting, you need fresh legs. And I promise that the strategies I've provided in this chapter will act as preventive medicine. You'll feel better and achieve more. Don't wait until your health fails and you're tackled short of your goals. Once you apply these strategies, you'll feel completely rejuvenated, and you'll be shocked by how much the quality of your life improves.

"Change is the essence of life. Be willing to sacrifice what you are for what you could become."

—TONY ROBBINS

10
WHERE YOU WILL GO FROM HERE

 "Unless commitment is made, there are only promises and hopes, but no plans."

—PETER F. DRUCKER

Congratulations, my friend—

just by reading this book, you've changed your life! You've taken a huge step toward world class. You've made an IMPACT. Before you move ahead, however, I'd like you to read the title of this final chapter again. I deliberately phrased it as a statement and not the more familiar question, "Where will you go from here?"

Where you go from here will not be a question, but a certainty. It will be a new journey. You've finished this book, done the hard work to complete the program, and given a 10-week jumpstart to your entire life, and now you have a choice to make. Follow the certainty of action—ready, fire, aim—the path that leads to accomplishment, transformation, and impact. Or follow the certainty of complacency—the path that leads backward to the life you left behind.

If you follow this program, you'll get results.

I know you will. But there is no finish line. Cherish and enjoy your accomplishments, but don't ever say, "Whew. I'm done." You're not done. You're never done. If you don't continue with this program, keep it in your life like the integral force it's been for 10 weeks, you'll end up like everyone else who has ever abandoned a plan after meeting a single goal. "Hey, I lost the weight I wanted to lose, I feel better, I don't need to do this anymore."

Wrong.

The biggest thing I asked you to do in this book

was commit. Now I'm telling you that if you do not remain committed to this program, all you have accomplished will disappear. Your weight will creep back up. Your old habits will return. And in the end, your body will decondition and compromise your health. We all have the power to take control of our health and fitness. I share this with you because of all the people who have inspired me. With all my might, I do not want you to become a statistic. Disease comes fast and hits hard. It's a lot like the two linebackers who ended my football career: Disease respects no rules, hits you when you're down, and always feels like a cheap shot.

The unfairness of the hit won't change the fact that you are down and hurt bad, perhaps permanently. I'm not putting these words on the page just to frighten you, or to preach. Diseases brought on by lifestyle are such a harsh and common reality in our society. And I've seen with my own eyes how disease can change your life literally in an instant.

I was 10 years old. My dad and I were on our way to watch a high school football game—a big one, my future high school, Brick, versus Toms River South. Just a massive Jersey rivalry. I was all jazzed about going and was bugging my dad in the parking lot outside the field because we were late.

"Come on, Dad, come on." My dad was 48, a big guy, 6-foot-3, 260 pounds, with the kind of electric personality that owned any room he stepped into. But now here he was, leaning against the bleachers, gripping his chest, unable to catch his breath. And I'm still tugging his arm, "Come on, Dad, come on, we're late!"

Finally he looks at me and says, "I'm having chest pains."

Two days later, he had triple bypass surgery.

My dad had always been an intense, hard-core, type-A guy, which fit him. Bigger than life. Fathered eight kids. As scary a day as that was for me— seeing this superhero stopped by some force I didn't understand—it was bigger for him, because it changed him. He went from a very driven personality to a more laid-back type B. It shifted his nature. As I grew up, he spent more time with me than he ever had. He attended every one of my practices and games in every sport—and I played all year round. That's a lot of time spent watching your son compete. Through him, I became an overachiever. In the process, I learned a lot of things, but maybe most important, I learned the value of hard work, and what it means to have someone believe in you.

"How you do anything, is how you do everything."

—TOM DAVIN

When I went away to college, I received a handwritten letter from my dad every single day. I'll say that again: every single day. Remember, e-mail didn't exist in the early '90s, so I would get a note along with something like a clipping from our local paper, the *Asbury Park Press*. For nearly 4 years of college. Imagine that commitment every day. He showed me what unconditional love was all about.

One morning when I was 20 and a senior at The College of William & Mary, I was pulled out of kinesiology class for an important phone call. My dad had just suffered a major heart attack. I was told to come right away. I flew home that afternoon. And for the first time, I understood the meaning of the word deathbed. But this man was my best friend, my hero, the man who wrote to me every single day. I felt that *IMPACT*, that anger and helplessness of receiving a cheap shot. I was being forced to accept something I didn't want to accept. The one thing I didn't want to lose was being taken from me. And as anyone who has ever experienced something similar with someone they love will tell you, all I could do was sit there and take it. My dad died the next day.

WHEN I RETURNED to campus 2 weeks later, a letter waited for me in my mailbox. He'd mailed it the day before the heart attack, the last letter I'd ever receive from him. It said, "You make me proud. Regardless of what you go into in the future, it doesn't matter as long as you do your best and make an impact in the world." I was blown away. I'd just buried my father, and he's writing to me about the rest of my life. Could he have known something bad was coming? He must have. But there he was, telling me to make an IMPACT while he'd just had the most incredible IMPACT on me. I had more of a dad in 20 years than most people get in a lifetime.

But here's the thing: He was 58 when he died. He'd never taken great care of himself; he carried a big belly, lived in an intense state of unresolved stress most of the time, didn't exercise regularly, ate poorly, all of it. He could very easily be alive today if he'd known more, done more.

This is what drives me every day. I can't change what happened. And I can't have what could have been. But I can help a whole lot of other people. I can make an IMPACT! That's my dad's legacy: Even though I've had decades of health and fitness training, education, experience, and the motivation to use it, my father taught me everything.

I ONCE READ a powerful poem called "The Dash," by Linda Ellis. Think about this: When you see someone's headstone, you see the year they were born and the year they died, like 1934–1992. But the dates aren't the important part. The most important part is that dash: What did you do between those dates, when you were alive and could make an impact on the people around you, on the world, on yourself? That's why the day you started this program and the day 10 weeks later when you finished don't necessarily matter. What did you do on the journey?

Now you have a new beginning. The day after you finish this program and decide how you'll go forward, your dash continues. How will *you* be better? How will *you* make an IMPACT?

You have to use the four Cs I talked about earlier in this book. They'll keep you focused. Commit to continuing the good work you started. Stay connected to the people you care about, and also to other people who have made an impact on their own lives with this program. Condition your body, mind, and spirit to carry you through this journey, to allow you to savor every last moment of it. I've set up an online playground and meeting place for you, **todddurkin.com**, where you'll find free tips and forums for visitors to keep each other informed and motivated. And of course, all of this will allow you to continue to create the life you want.

"*Champions know that there is a difference between interest and commitment. When you're interested in something, you do it only when circumstances permit. When you're committed to something, you accept no excuses, only results!*"

—AUTHOR UNKNOWN

Before you go, however, I have one last exercise for you. An extra 1 percent before you hit the showers. A little "and then some."

You're going to make another decree.

This one will be even more impactful than your first decree, which was all about a 10-week quest for transformation. Now I want you to decree what the next year will look like after you've experienced it.

See, I've given you the tools—heck, an entire toolbox!—of transformation. You have know-how, motivation, and accountability. Now you have to think bigger. A whole year! That's exciting. That's powerful. Imagine what you could accomplish in a year.

THERE'S ONE THING about achieving health and fitness that I think goes unspoken and unwritten too often: We know what we have to do.

I've given you an entire book of new tools, motivation, and a recipe to give you exactly what you need to do to take control of your life. And now that you've read *The IMPACT! Body Plan* and have this new set of tools in your hand, I say it again: You know what you have to do.

Commit, connect, condition, create.

Ready, fire, aim.

10 in—10 out.

And then some!

It's your time now. You have the game plan. You know your opponent. Maybe you have some fear— fear of change, fear of commitment, fear that you might actually discover how powerful you really are and all your comforting excuses will have to be cast aside. That is scary. But fear is okay as long as you use it. Not many people do. There are too many people letting fear guide them, too many scared people feeling trapped in lives that seem more like prison than living. Well, friends, lace up yo ur shoes and start. That's all you have to do. You will discover an energy shift that changes your health, your performance, your career, your relationships, and your appetite for both food and life itself. Tie your shoes. Commit. Move.

You'll sometimes have bad days. You'll sometimes meet with adversity. You'll sometimes feel resistance from your own brain and receive resistance from everyone and everything else in your life. That's why I've said from the very beginning that everyone has to train like a professional athlete. Because pros train with intensity and consistency. They attack any and all obstacles because they want to win so badly they can taste the champagne victory shower. Their minds and bodies are strong, and they never quit, not even on the worst day.

Pros specialize in changing momentum. Watch any sport, from football to golf to tennis, and you see constant changes in momentum because neither side will quit. Fight for your momentum. Simply taking action gives you a huge momentum shift that you can build on. You can do it. 10 in—10 out.

So . . . I've said all I can say to you, given you all the knowledge you need. Now you need to deliver for yourself. You need *you*. What will your game-changing move be? Quit? Or fight like a champion? IMPACT? Or no impact? Life? Or death?

Choose now. Your life depends on it.

WRITE YOUR DECREE *for the next 365 days*

Assess the same areas as before, but go bigger: How will I be transformed? What new and amazing things will I try? How will I make an impact on myself and those I care about? How have my goals grown and expanded? How have I laid the groundwork for my legacy? If the last day of this year happened to be my last day of all, what would my dash be?

Make your decree now. Remember to write it as if it has already happened. You can start by saying, "I am so grateful and happy now that . . . " Then write as if you are looking back 1 year from now and showing gratitude for all that has been achieved. Take your time with it. Hone it. Make it count. When it's complete, condense it down so that it fits on an index card, just as you did with your first decree, back in Chapter 3. Select words that move and inspire you. Read your card every morning for the next 365 days. Stay on the path. Make a difference for yourself and others. Make an IMPACT.

IMPACT, baby . . .
AND THEN SOME!

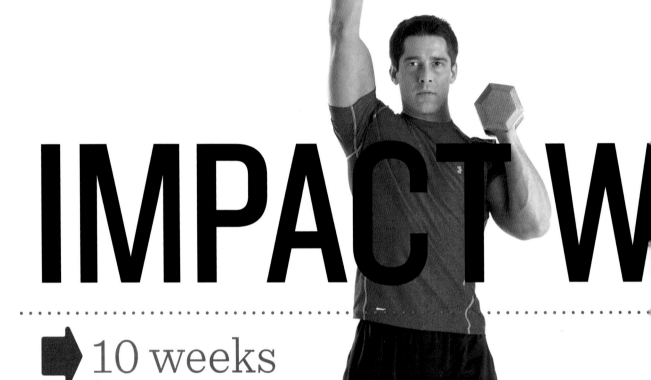

IMPACT W

➡ 10 weeks

KEY

➡ 1 x 15 | p. 232

indicates 1 set
of 15 reps

where to find
a description
of the exercise

KB	**DB**	**SB**	**SC**	**MB**
kettlebell	dumbbell	Superband	Sports Cord	medicine ball

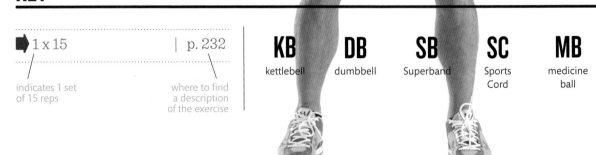

ORKOUTS

A Quick-Start Guide

Use this overview as a performance guide for the next 10 weeks. This is your game plan, while the exercises in the back of the book are your playbook. You need both.

Stage I
TOTAL-BODY WORKOUTS

Weeks 1–3
TRAINING CAMP

Three days per week you'll perform resistance (strength) training using all seven phases of the Matrix.

One day a week your workout will be boot camp–style.

You can perform additional cardio 1 or 2 days a week.

You'll take at least 1 day off from all exercise each week.

Stage II
SPLIT-FUSION WORKOUTS

Weeks 4–7
IN SEASON

Stage III
SPLIT-FUSION WORKOUTS

Weeks 8–10
THE PLAYOFFS

You'll do one total-body workout per week.

You'll have 1 day of predominantly lower-body and core work.

One day will focus on your upper body and core.

You'll do 1 day of boot camp total-body conditioning using body-weight exercises.

You can perform additional cardio 1 or 2 days a week.

You'll take at least 1 day off from all exercise each week.

WEEK 1

TOTAL-BODY WORKOUT

Every workout begins with a thorough dynamic warmup and exercises for your joints that is followed by resistance (strength) training using a high-intensity, high-tempo interval style. These workouts include all seven phases of the Matrix (dynamic warmup, joint integrity, core conditioning, power and plyometrics, strength and conditioning, movement training, and flexibility). A typical station will consist of a lower-body exercise, a push exercise, and a pull exercise.

1 THE DYNAMIC WARMUP

JUMPING JACK
10 reps

GATE SWING
10 reps

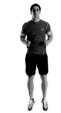
POGO HOP
20 reps

SEAL JACK
10 reps

BODYWEIGHT SQUAT
10 reps

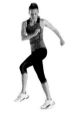
SIDE LUNGE
10 reps / side

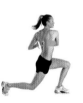
LUNGE AND ROTATE
10 reps / side

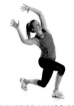
REVERSE LUNGE AND REACH OVER TOP
5 reps / side

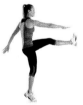
CARIOCA
10 yards

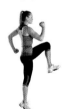
SKIPPING FORWARD
10 yards

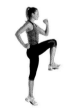
SKIPPING BACKWARD
10 yards

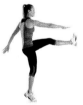
FRANKENSTEIN WALK
10 yards

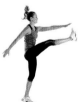
FRANKENSTEIN SKIP
10 yards

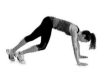
INCHWORM
5–10 reps

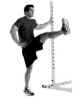
HIP SWING
10 reps / leg

2 JOINT INTEGRITY

Rest approximately 30 seconds between exercises.

MON Hips

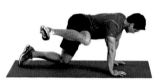

DIRTY DOG
➡ 1 x 15 / leg | p. 226

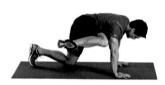

HORSEBACK RIDING
➡ 1 x 10 / leg | p. 227

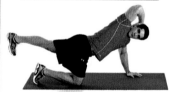

BIRD DOG AND ROTATE
➡ 1 x 10 / side | p. 226

WED Shoulders

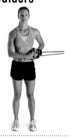

SC EXTERNAL ROTATION
➡ 1 x 15 / arm | p. 241

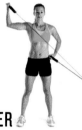

SC HITCHHIKER
➡ 1 x 15 / arm | p. 242

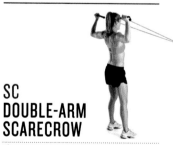

SC DOUBLE-ARM SCARECROW
➡ 1 x 15 | p. 242

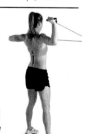

SC SINGLE-ARM SCARECROW
➡ 1 x max / arm | p. 241

FRI Balance / barefoot

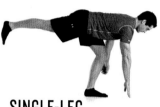

SINGLE-LEG BALANCE TOUCH
➡ 1 x 10 / leg | p. 225

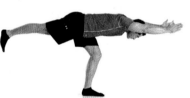

SINGLE-LEG BALANCE REACH-FORWARD
➡ 1 x 10 / leg | p. 230

WEEK 1 MON

TOTAL-BODY WORKOUT

Perform all exercises with the same number as a circuit—that is, one set of all exercises in the circuit (1a, 1b, 1c)—and then repeat. Move on to the next series of exercises once all sets are complete.

3 CORE

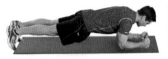

1 HOVER PLANK
➧ 1 x 30 seconds | p. 228

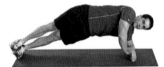

2 HIPUP
➧ 1 x 15 / side | p. 231

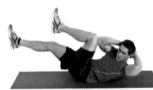

3 BICYCLE AND ROTATE
➧ 2 x max | p. 228

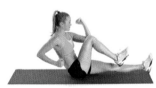

4 RUNNING-MAN SITUP
➧ 1 x max | p. 230

4 STRENGTH

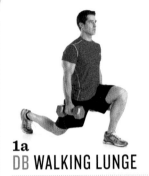

1a DB WALKING LUNGE
➧ 2 x 20 | p. 260

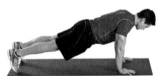

1b PUSHUP
➧ 2 x 20 | p. 229

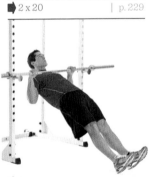

1c RACK ROW
➧ 2 x 10–15 | p. 235

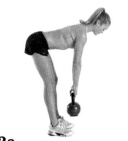

2a
KB DOUBLE-LEG ROMANIAN DEADLIFT

➡ 2 x 12 | p. 252

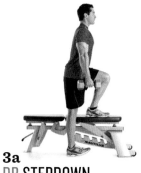

3a
DB STEPDOWN

➡ 2 x 10 / leg | p. 264

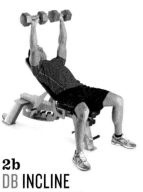

2b
DB INCLINE BENCH PRESS

➡ 2 x 15 | p. 263

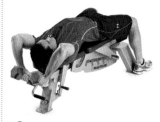

3b
DB ROLLING TRICEPS SUPERSET

➡ 2 x 10 | p. 263

2c
SB ½-KNEELING PULLDOWN

➡ 2 x 10–15 | p. 247

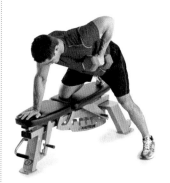

3c
DB SINGLE-ARM ROW

➡ 2 x 12 / arm | p. 261

IMPACT DICTIONARY

Grand Finale Conditioning

At the end of many workouts, you'll see "grand finale conditioning" (GFC). I love to design my workouts with some final conditioning where you can leave everything behind and empty the tank. This is a game changer, my friends.

You'll have GFC on Mondays, Thursdays, and Saturdays after boot camp. You can use a treadmill, bike, elliptical trainer, rower, or VersaClimber, or you can run or power walk outside or jump rope. The rules are simple: Start slowly, gradually increase your speed, and challenge yourself appropriately. Push yourself as hard as you want here. The more you challenge yourself, the better your results will be.

GRAND FINALE
CONDITIONING
after workout

Treadmill, bike, jumping rope, boxing, etc.
**30 SECONDS ON
30–60 SECONDS OFF**

3 sets

WEEK 1
WED

TOTAL-BODY WORKOUT

3 CORE

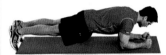

1
HOVER PLANK
➡ 1 x 30 seconds | p. 228

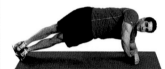

2
HIPUP
➡ 1 x 15 / side | p. 231

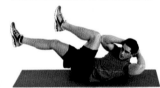

3
BICYCLE AND ROTATE
➡ 2 x max | p. 228

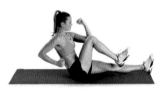

4
RUNNING-MAN SITUP
➡ 1 x max | p. 230

4 STRENGTH

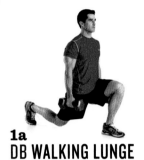

1a
DB WALKING LUNGE
➡ 2 x 20 | p. 260

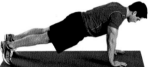

1b
PUSHUP
➡ 2 x 20 | p. 229

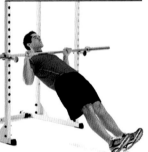

1c
RACK ROW
➡ 2 x 10–15 | p. 235

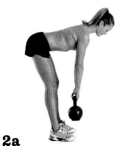

2a
KB DOUBLE-LEG
ROMANIAN DEADLIFT
➡ 2 x 12 | p. 252

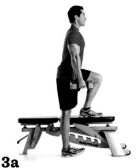

3a
DB STEPDOWN
➡ 2 x 10 / leg | p. 264

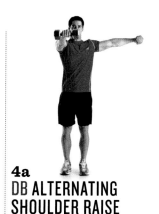

4a
DB ALTERNATING
SHOULDER RAISE
➡ 2 x 8 / arm | p. 258

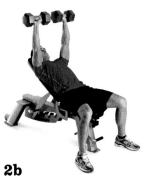

2b
DB INCLINE
BENCH PRESS
➡ 2 x 15 | p. 263

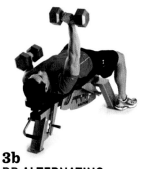

3b
DB ALTERNATING
BENCH PRESS
➡ 2 x 10 / arm | p. 262

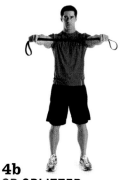

4b
SB SPLITTER
➡ 2 x 15 | p. 242

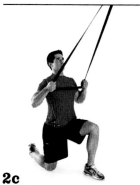

2c
SB ½-KNEELING
PULLDOWN
➡ 2 x 12–15 | p. 247

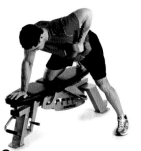

3c
DB SINGLE-ARM ROW
➡ 2 x 12 | p. 261

GRAND FINALE
CONDITIONING
after workout

Treadmill, bike, jumping
rope, boxing, etc.
**30 SECONDS ON
30–60 SECONDS OFF**

3 sets

WEEK 1 FRI

TOTAL-BODY WORKOUT

3 CORE

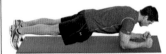

1
HOVER PLANK

➡ 1 x 30 seconds | p. 228

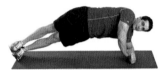

2
HIPUP

➡ 1 x 15 / side | p. 231

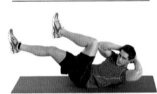

3
BICYCLE AND ROTATE

➡ 2 x max | p. 228

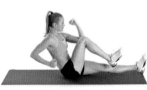

4
RUNNING-MAN SITUP

➡ 1 x max | p. 230

4 STRENGTH

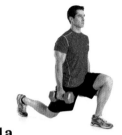

1a
DB WALKING LUNGE

➡ 2 x 20 | p. 260

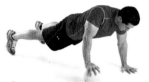

1b
MB SINGLE-ARM PUSHUP

➡ 2 x 20 | p. 248

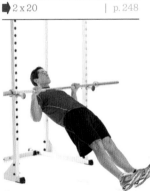

1c
RACK ROW

➡ 2 x 10–15 | p. 235

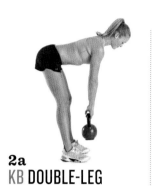

2a
KB DOUBLE-LEG
ROMANIAN DEADLIFT

➡ 2 x 12 | p. 252

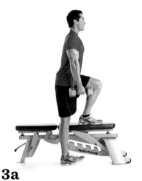

3a
DB STEPDOWN

➡ 2 x 10 / leg | p. 264

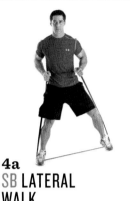

4a
SB LATERAL
WALK

➡ 2 x 15 / side | p. 243

GRAND FINALE
CONDITIONING
after workout

Treadmill, bike, jumping
rope, boxing, etc.
**30 SECONDS ON
30–60 SECONDS OFF**

3 sets

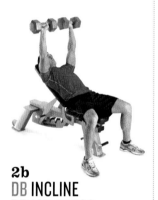

2b
DB INCLINE
BENCH PRESS

➡ 2 x 15 | p. 263

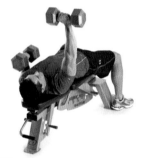

3b
DB ALTERNATING
BENCH PRESS

➡ 2 x 10 / arm | p. 262

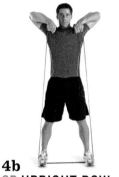

4b
SB UPRIGHT ROW

➡ 2 x 15 | p. 243

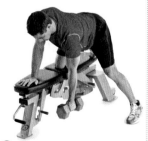

2c
SB ½-KNEELING
PULLDOWN

➡ 2 x 10–15 | p. 247

3c
DB SINGLE-ARM ROW

➡ 2 x 12 / arm | p. 261

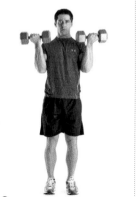

4c
DB BICEPS CURL

➡ 2 x 15 | p. 257

1-3

BOOT CAMP

This boot camp workout requires no equipment—just your body and a bench. As with every workout, the key is tempo. Try to move fast, and rest as little as possible between exercises, aiming for 30 to 60 seconds at most. Rest 1 to 2 minutes between circuits.

Warmup:

 WALK OR JOG FOR 5–10 MINUTES

CIRCUIT 1

Repeat the circuit 2 times. Then run for 3–5 minutes.

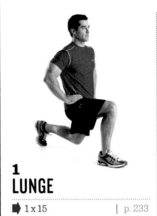

1
LUNGE

➡ 1 x 15 | p. 233

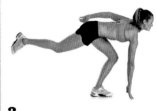

3
SINGLE-LEG BALANCE TOUCH

➡ 1 x 10 / side | p. 225

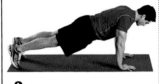

2
PUSHUP

➡ 1 x 15 | p. 229

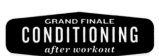

GRAND FINALE
CONDITIONING
after workout

Sprint
30 SECONDS ON
60 SECONDS OFF
2–3 sets

CIRCUIT 2

Repeat the circuit 2 times. Then run for 3–5 minutes.

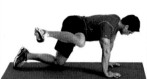

1
DIRTY DOG

➡ 1 x 15 / leg | p. 226

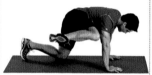

2
HORSEBACK RIDING

➡ 1 x 10 / leg | p. 227

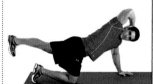

3
BIRD DOG AND ROTATE

➡ 1 x 10 / side | p. 226

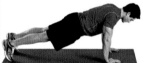

4
PUSHUP

➡ 1 x 15 | p. 229

CIRCUIT 3

Repeat circuit 2 times.

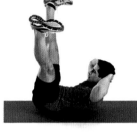

1
HELLO DOLLY

➡ 1 x 20 | p. 232

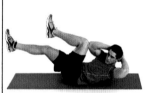

2
BICYCLE AND ROTATE

➡ 1 x max | p. 228

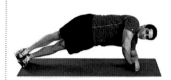

3
HIPUP

➡ 1 x 20 | p. 231

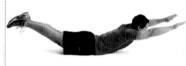

4
SUPERMAN

➡ 1 x 15 | p. 233

IN THE TRENCHES
GFCs

You might think that grand finale conditioning is a favorite of my athletes (and it is), but it's my regulars who love this end-of-training challenge the most. One of my longtime clients, Mary McKay, has turned GFCs into her own personal competition. At the end of her workouts, she runs on a treadmill and tests how fast she can run.

After a 2-minute warmup jogging at 7 miles per hour, Mary starts to pick up the pace. She'll sprint for 1 minute and then rest for the same amount of time. Mary continues to pick up the pace after each break, matching her rest period to her running time (for instance, 45 seconds of running and 45 seconds of rest). Her personal best is a 30-second sprint at 12 miles per hour followed by a mere 30-second break. Can you match her intensity?

WEEK 2
TRAINING CAMP

TOTAL-BODY WORKOUT

1 THE DYNAMIC WARMUP

Follow the instructions from page 114, or perform each movement for 10 to 20 seconds.

1 JUMPING JACK	7 LUNGE & ROTATE	12 FRANKENSTEIN WALK
2 GATE SWING	8 REVERSE LUNGE & REACH OVER TOP	13 FRANKENSTEIN SKIP
3 POGO HOP	9 CARIOCA	14 INCHWORM
4 SEAL JACK	10 SKIPPING FORWARD	15 HIP SWING
5 BODY-WEIGHT SQUAT	11 SKIPPING BACKWARD	
6 SIDE LUNGE		

2 JOINT INTEGRITY

Rest approximately 30 seconds between exercises.

MON Hips

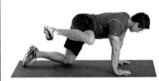

1
DIRTY DOG
➡ 1 x 15 / leg | p. 226

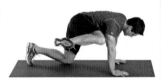

2
HORSEBACK RIDING
➡ 1 x 10 / leg | p. 227

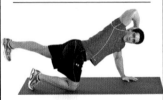

3
BIRD DOG AND ROTATE
➡ 1 x 10 / side | p. 226

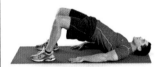

4
HIP BRIDGE
➡ 1 x 10 | p. 231

WED Shoulders

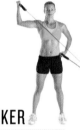

1
SC EXTERNAL ROTATION
➡ 1 x 15 / arm | p. 241

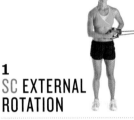

2
SB HITCHHIKER
➡ 1 x 15 / arm | p. 242

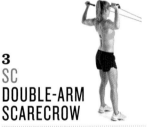

3
SC DOUBLE-ARM SCARECROW
➡ 1 x 15 | p. 242

4
SC SINGLE-ARM SCARECROW
➡ 1 x 15 / arm | p. 241

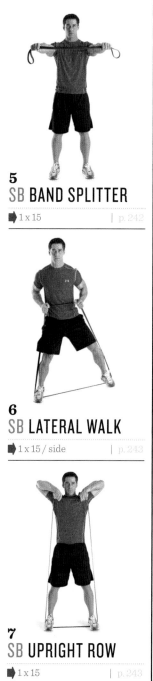

5
SB BAND SPLITTER
➡ 1 x 15 | p. 242

6
SB LATERAL WALK
➡ 1 x 15 / side | p. 243

7
SB UPRIGHT ROW
➡ 1 x 15 | p. 243

FRI
Balance / barefoot

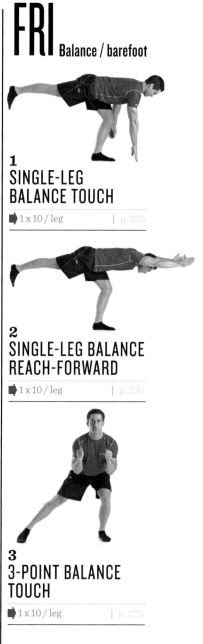

1
SINGLE-LEG BALANCE TOUCH
➡ 1 x 10 / leg | p. 225

2
SINGLE-LEG BALANCE REACH-FORWARD
➡ 1 x 10 / leg | p. 230

3
3-POINT BALANCE TOUCH
➡ 1 x 10 / leg | p. 225

AND THEN SOME

Try Barefoot Training

Barefoot training during the dynamic warmup and the balance portion of joint integrity is a great way to work the foundation of your body: your feet. By taking off your shoes and making your feet work more, you'll strengthen all the small intrinsic muscles in your feet and lower legs. This can help prevent injuries such as plantar fasciitis and shinsplints, as well as so many other ailments of the body. Strong feet build a stronger structure, which helps protect your knees, your hips, and even your lower back. This helps ensure a strong foundation for your kinetic chain. Feel free to train in your bare feet for any of the balance training in the IMPACT program.

WEEK 2 MON

TRAINING CAMP

TOTAL-BODY WORKOUT

3 CORE

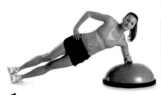

1
BOSU HIPUP

➡ 1 x 10 / side | p. 237

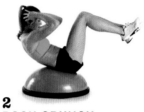

2
BOSU CRUNCH AND KICK

➡ 1 x 15 | p. 237

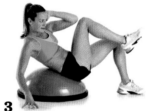

3
BOSU OPPOSITE ELBOW AND KNEE

➡ 1 x 10 / side | p. 240

4 STRENGTH

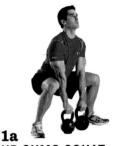

1a
KB SUMO SQUAT

➡ 2 x 10 | p. 253

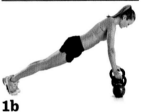

1b
KB PUSHUP

➡ 2 x 10 | p. 250

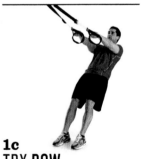

1c
TRX ROW

➡ 2 x 15 | p. 255

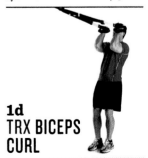

1d
TRX BICEPS CURL

➡ 2 x 10 | p. 257

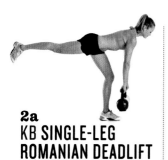

2a
KB SINGLE-LEG ROMANIAN DEADLIFT
➡ 2 x 8 / leg | p. 252

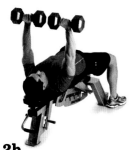

2b
DB BENCH PRESS
➡ 2 x 8 | p. 262

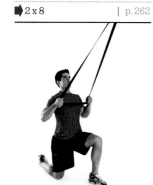

2c
SB ½-KNEELING PULLDOWN
➡ 2 x 10–15 | p. 247

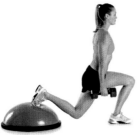

3a
BOSU BULGARIAN LUNGE
➡ 2 x 15 | p. 239

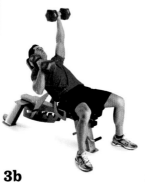

3b
DB INCLINE ALTERNATING BENCH PRESS
➡ 2 x 10 / arm | p. 263

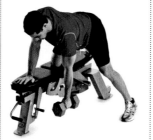

3c
DB SINGLE-ARM ROW
➡ 2 x 12 / arm | p. 261

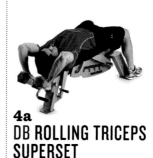

4a
DB ROLLING TRICEPS SUPERSET
➡ 2–3 x 10 | p. 263

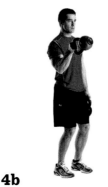

4b
KB ALTERNATING HAMMER CURL
➡ 2–3 x 10 | p. 253

GRAND FINALE
CONDITIONING
after workout

Treadmill, bike, jumping rope, boxing, etc.
**30 SECONDS ON
30–45 SECONDS OFF**
4 sets

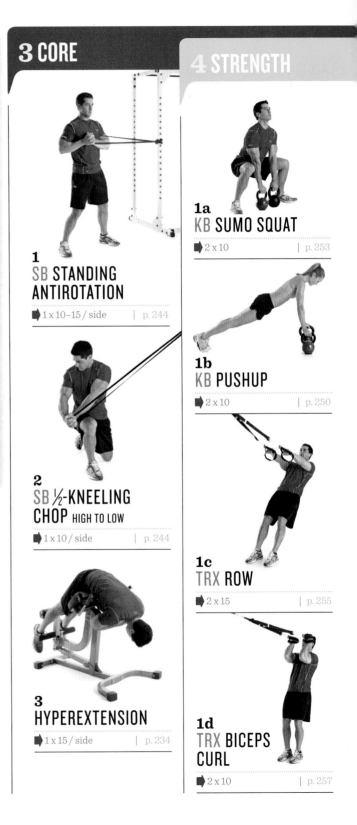

WEEK 2 WED

TRAINING CAMP

TOTAL-BODY WORKOUT

3 CORE

1
SB STANDING ANTIROTATION
➡ 1 x 10–15 / side | p. 244

2
SB ½-KNEELING CHOP HIGH TO LOW
➡ 1 x 10 / side | p. 244

3
HYPEREXTENSION
➡ 1 x 15 / side | p. 234

4 STRENGTH

1a
KB SUMO SQUAT
➡ 2 x 10 | p. 253

1b
KB PUSHUP
➡ 2 x 10 | p. 250

1c
TRX ROW
➡ 2 x 15 | p. 255

1d
TRX BICEPS CURL
➡ 2 x 10 | p. 257

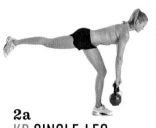

2a
KB SINGLE-LEG ROMANIAN DEADLIFT

➡ 2 x 8 / leg | p. 252

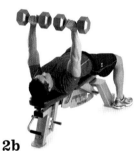

2b
DB BENCH PRESS

➡ 2 x 8 | p. 262

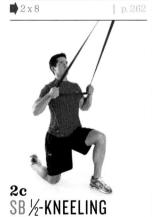

2c
SB ½-KNEELING PULLDOWN

➡ 2 x 10–15 | p. 247

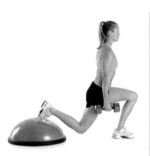

3a
BOSU BULGARIAN LUNGE

➡ 2 x 15 | p. 239

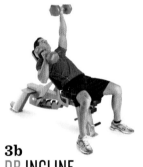

3b
DB INCLINE ALTERNATING BENCH PRESS

➡ 2 x 10 / arm | p. 263

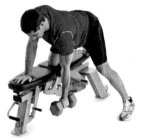

3c
DB SINGLE-ARM ROW

➡ 2 x 12 / arm | p. 261

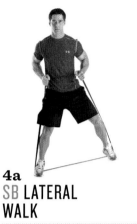

4a
SB LATERAL WALK

➡ 2 x 15 | p. 243

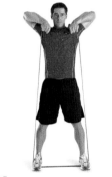

4b
SB UPRIGHT ROW

➡ 2 x 15 | p. 243

GRAND FINALE
CONDITIONING
after workout

Treadmill, bike, jumping rope, boxing, etc.
**30 SECONDS ON
30–45 SECONDS OFF**
4 sets

WEEK 2 FRI

TRAINING CAMP

TOTAL-BODY WORKOUT

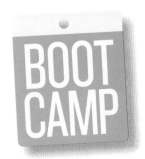

BOOT CAMP

Perform Saturday's boot camp using the workout on page 122.

3 CORE

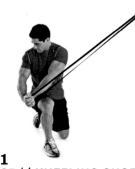

1
SB ½-KNEELING CHOP
HIGH TO LOW

➡ 1 x 10 / side | p. 244

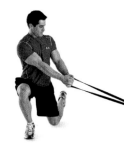

2
SB ½-KNEELING LIFTS
LOW TO HIGH

➡ 1 x 10 / side | p. 244

4 STRENGTH

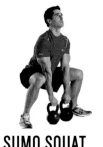

1a
KB SUMO SQUAT

➡ 2 x 10 | p. 253

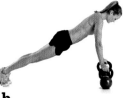

1b
KB PUSHUP

➡ 2 x 10 | p. 250

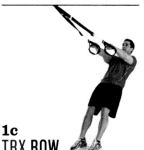

1c
TRX ROW

➡ 2 x 15 | p. 255

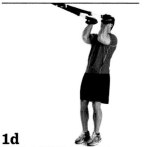

1d
TRX BICEPS CURL

➡ 2 x 10 | p. 257

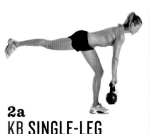

2a
KB SINGLE-LEG
ROMANIAN DEADLIFT
➡ 2 x 8 / leg　　　　| p. 252

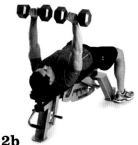

2b
DB BENCH PRESS
➡ 2 x 8　　　　| p. 262

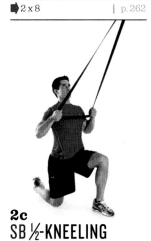

2c
SB ½-KNEELING
PULLDOWN
➡ 2 x 10–15　　　　| p. 247

3a
BOSU BULGARIAN
LUNGE
➡ 2 x 15 / leg　　　　| p. 239

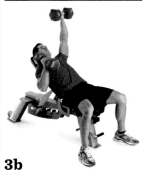

3b
DB INCLINE
ALTERNATING
BENCH PRESS
➡ 2 x 10 / arm　　　　| p. 263

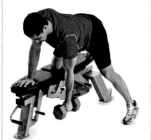

3c
DB SINGLE-ARM ROW
➡ 2 x 12 / arm　　　　| p. 261

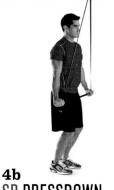

4a
SB OVERHEAD
TRICEPS EXTENSION
➡ 2 x 10–15　　　　| p. 246

4b
SB PRESSDOWN
➡ 2 x 10–15　　　　| p. 246

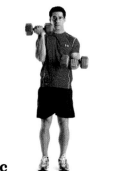

4c
BICEPS 10/10/10
➡ 2 sets　　　　| p. 262

GRAND FINALE
CONDITIONING
after workout

Treadmill, bike, jumping
rope, boxing, etc.
**30 SECONDS ON
30–45 SECONDS OFF**
4 sets

WEEK 3

TRAINING CAMP

TOTAL-BODY WORKOUT

1 THE DYNAMIC WARMUP

Follow the instructions from page 114,
or perform each movement for 10 to 20 seconds.

1 JUMPING JACK	7 LUNGE & ROTATE	12 FRANKENSTEIN WALK
2 GATE SWING	8 REVERSE LUNGE & REACH OVER TOP	13 FRANKENSTEIN SKIP
3 POGO HOP	9 CARIOCA	14 INCHWORM
4 SEAL JACK	10 SKIPPING FORWARD	15 HIP SWING
5 BODY-WEIGHT SQUAT	11 SKIPPING BACKWARD	
6 SIDE LUNGE		

2 JOINT INTEGRITY

Rest approximately 30 seconds between exercises.

MON Hips

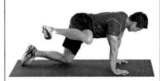

**1
DIRTY DOG**

➡ 2 x 15 / leg | p. 226

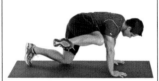

**2
HORSEBACK RIDING**

➡ 2 x 10 / leg | p. 227

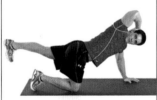

**3
BIRD DOG AND ROTATE**

➡ 2 x 10 / side | p. 226

WED Shoulders

**1
SC EXTERNAL ROTATION**

➡ 1 x 15 / arm | p. 241

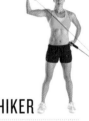

**2
SC HITCHHIKER**

➡ 1 x 10 / arm | p. 242

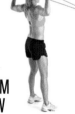

**3
SB DOUBLE-ARM SCARECROW**

➡ 1 x 10 | p. 242

**4
SB SINGLE-ARM SCARECROW**

➡ 1 x 10 / arm | p. 241

FRI Balance

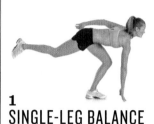

1
SINGLE-LEG BALANCE TOUCH

➡ 1 x 10 / leg | p. 225

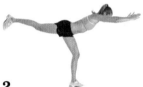

2
SINGLE-LEG BALANCE REACH-FORWARD

➡ 1 x 10 / leg | p. 230

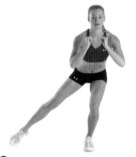

3
3-POINT BALANCE TOUCH

➡ 1 x 10 / leg | p. 225

IMPACT DICTIONARY

Intuitive Training

The IMPACT workouts are a structured blueprint to help you improve your body and overall health. You'll find reps, sets, and rest intervals. But if you look closely, sometimes the rep ranges and sets vary without a fixed recommendation. That's intentional. I want to teach you to listen to your body and train intuitively. There are days when you'll feel great and want to push forward. Do it. Other times you might need to hold back. But when you learn to decipher what your body wants, you can bend the rules a little bit. Do a few extra reps. Crank out another set. Just make sure that you're listening to your body, pushing forward when you can, and reining back when it's needed. Listen to that body and play!

No matter what, always show up for a workout and do something. Sometimes just getting the engine revved for 10 minutes will help you get your mind right for the day and make you feel better. Even if it's not your best workout, keep on pushing yourself to make exercise a part of your life. In the end, just making that effort can be the difference between success and failure.

WEEK 3 MON

TRAINING CAMP

TOTAL-BODY WORKOUT

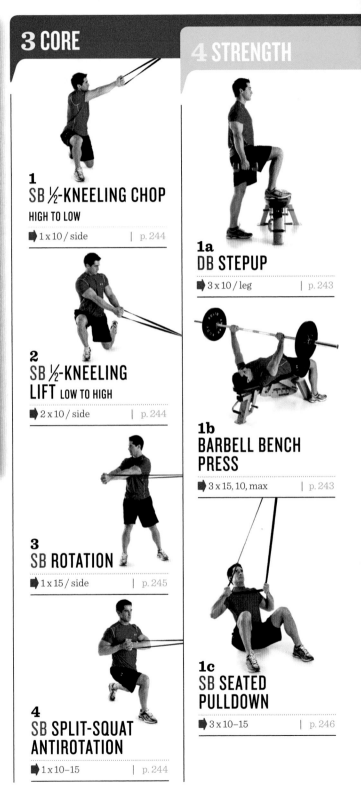

3 CORE

1
SB ½-KNEELING CHOP
HIGH TO LOW

➡ 1 x 10 / side | p. 244

2
SB ½-KNEELING LIFT **LOW TO HIGH**

➡ 2 x 10 / side | p. 244

3
SB ROTATION

➡ 1 x 15 / side | p. 245

4
SB SPLIT-SQUAT ANTIROTATION

➡ 1 x 10–15 | p. 244

4 STRENGTH

1a
DB STEPUP

➡ 3 x 10 / leg | p. 243

1b
BARBELL BENCH PRESS

➡ 3 x 15, 10, max | p. 243

1c
SB SEATED PULLDOWN

➡ 3 x 10–15 | p. 246

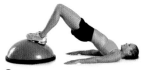

2a
BOSU HIP BRIDGE

➡ 2 x 15 | p. 238

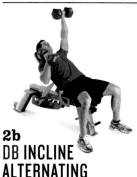

2b
DB INCLINE ALTERNATING BENCH PRESS

➡ 2 x 15 / arm | p. 263

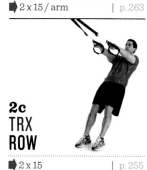

2c
TRX ROW

➡ 2 x 15 | p. 255

2d
TRX BICEPS CURL

➡ 2 x 15 | p. 257

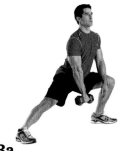

3a
DB SIDE LUNGE

➡ 2 x 8 / side | p. 261

3b
BURPEE

➡ 2 x 10 | p. 229

3c
SB SQUAT AND SINGLE-ARM ROW AND ROTATE

➡ 2 x 10 / arm | p. 247

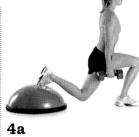

4a
BOSU BULGARIAN LUNGE

➡ 2 x 10 / leg | p. 239

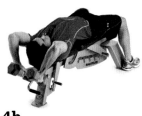
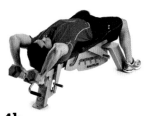

4b
DB ROLLING TRICEPS SUPERSET

➡ 2 x 10–15 | p. 263

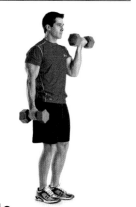

4c
DB ALTERNATING BICEPS CURL

➡ 2 x 8–10 / arm | p. 258

GRAND FINALE
CONDITIONING
after workout

Treadmill, bike, jumping rope, boxing, etc.

**30 SECONDS ON
30 SECONDS OFF**

5 sets

WEEK 3 WED

TRAINING CAMP

TOTAL-BODY WORKOUT

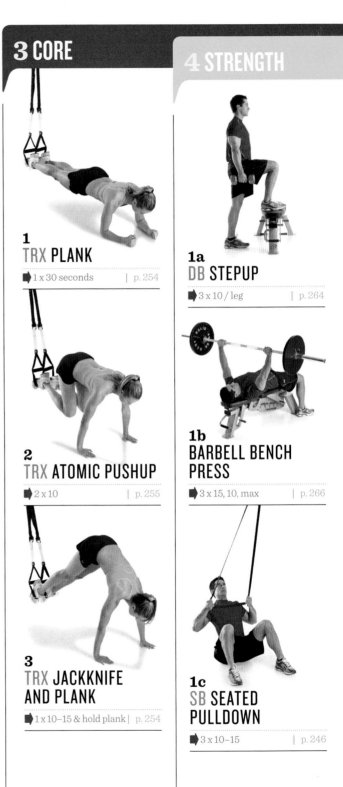

3 CORE

1
TRX PLANK
➡ 1 x 30 seconds | p. 254

2
TRX ATOMIC PUSHUP
➡ 2 x 10 | p. 255

3
TRX JACKKNIFE AND PLANK
➡ 1 x 10–15 & hold plank | p. 254

4 STRENGTH

1a
DB STEPUP
➡ 3 x 10 / leg | p. 264

1b
BARBELL BENCH PRESS
➡ 3 x 15, 10, max | p. 266

1c
SB SEATED PULLDOWN
➡ 3 x 10–15 | p. 246

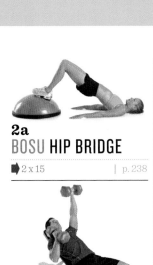

2a
BOSU HIP BRIDGE

➡ 2 x 15 | p. 238

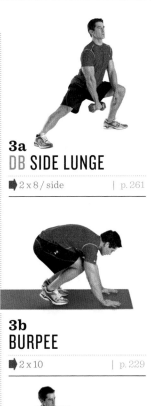

3a
DB SIDE LUNGE

➡ 2 x 8 / side | p. 261

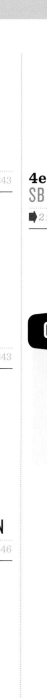

4a
SB LATERAL WALK

➡ 2 x 15 / side | p. 243

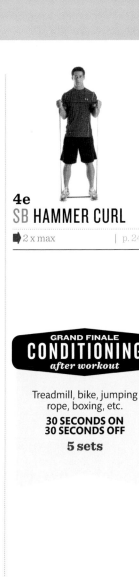

4e
SB HAMMER CURL

➡ 2 x max | p. 243

2b
DB INCLINE
ALTERNATING
BENCH PRESS

➡ 2 x 15 / arm | p. 263

3b
BURPEE

➡ 2 x 10 | p. 229

4b
SB UPRIGHT ROW

➡ 2 x 15 | p. 243

GRAND FINALE
CONDITIONING
after workout

Treadmill, bike, jumping
rope, boxing, etc.
**30 SECONDS ON
30 SECONDS OFF**

5 sets

2c
TRX ROW

➡ 2 x 15 | p. 255

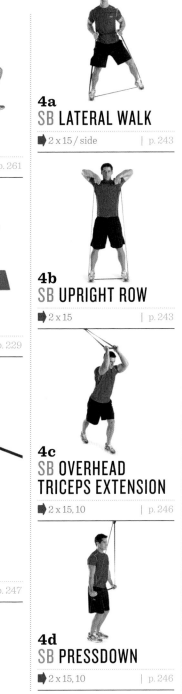

4c
SB OVERHEAD
TRICEPS EXTENSION

➡ 2 x 15, 10 | p. 246

3c
SB SQUAT AND
SINGLE-ARM ROW
AND ROTATE

➡ 2 x 10 / arm | p. 247

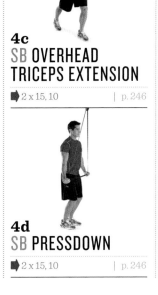

2d
TRX BICEPS CURL

➡ 2 x 15 | p. 257

4d
SB PRESSDOWN

➡ 2 x 15, 10 | p. 246

WEEK 3 FRI

TRAINING CAMP

TOTAL-BODY WORKOUT

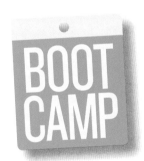

BOOT CAMP

Perform Saturday's boot camp using the workout on page 122.

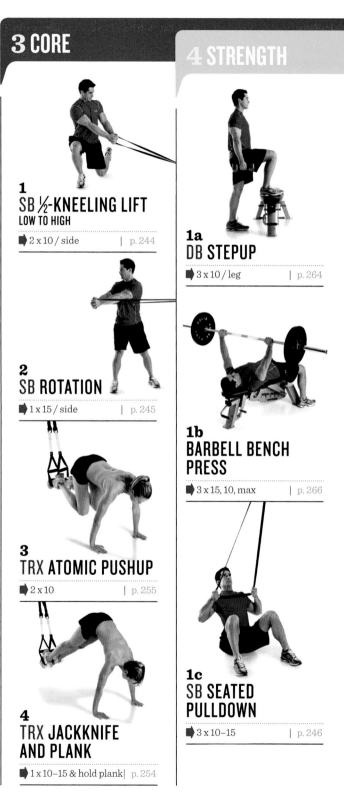

3 CORE

1
SB ½-KNEELING LIFT
LOW TO HIGH

➡ 2 x 10 / side | p. 244

2
SB ROTATION

➡ 1 x 15 / side | p. 245

3
TRX ATOMIC PUSHUP

➡ 2 x 10 | p. 255

4
TRX JACKKNIFE AND PLANK

➡ 1 x 10–15 & hold plank | p. 254

4 STRENGTH

1a
DB STEPUP

➡ 3 x 10 / leg | p. 264

1b
BARBELL BENCH PRESS

➡ 3 x 15, 10, max | p. 266

1c
SB SEATED PULLDOWN

➡ 3 x 10–15 | p. 246

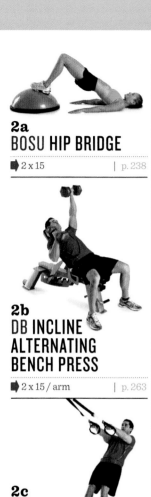

2a
BOSU HIP BRIDGE

➡ 2 x 15 | p. 238

2b
DB INCLINE ALTERNATING BENCH PRESS

➡ 2 x 15 / arm | p. 263

2c
TRX ROW

➡ 2 x 15 | p. 255

2d
TRX BICEPS CURL

➡ 2 x 15 | p. 257

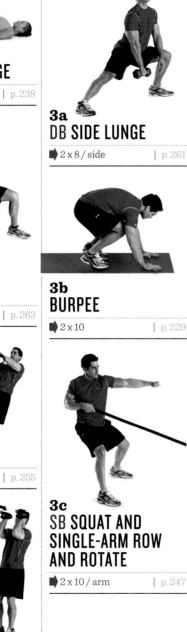

3a
DB SIDE LUNGE

➡ 2 x 8 / side | p. 261

3b
BURPEE

➡ 2 x 10 | p. 229

3c
SB SQUAT AND SINGLE-ARM ROW AND ROTATE

➡ 2 x 10 / arm | p. 247

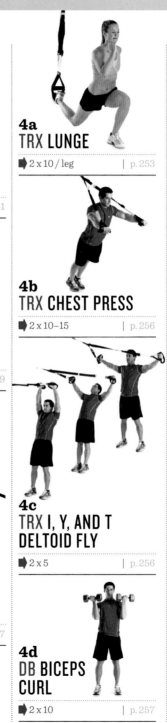

4a
TRX LUNGE

➡ 2 x 10 / leg | p. 253

4b
TRX CHEST PRESS

➡ 2 x 10–15 | p. 256

4c
TRX I, Y, AND T DELTOID FLY

➡ 2 x 5 | p. 256

4d
DB BICEPS CURL

➡ 2 x 10 | p. 257

GRAND FINALE
CONDITIONING
after workout

Treadmill, bike, jumping rope, boxing, etc.
**30 SECONDS ON
30 SECONDS OFF**
5 sets

WEEK 4 MON

IN SEASON

PLYOMETRICS & POWER

1 THE DYNAMIC WARMUP

1 JUMPING JACK	7 LUNGE & ROTATE	12 SKIPPING BACKWARD
2 GATE SWING	8 REVERSE LUNGE & REACH OVER TOP	13 FRANKENSTEIN WALK
3 POGO HOP	9 CARIOCA	14 FRANKENSTEIN SKIP
4 SEAL JACK	10 LIZARD CRAWL	15 INCHWORM
5 BODYWEIGHT SQUAT	11 SKIPPING FORWARD	16 HIP SWING
6 SIDE LUNGE		*new!*

2 JOINT INTEGRITY

Rest approximately 30 seconds between exercises.

Hips + Shoulders

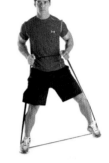

1
DIRTY DOG

➡ 2 x 15 / leg | p. 226

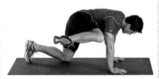

2
HORSEBACK RIDING

➡ 1 x 10 / leg | p. 227

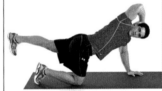

3
BIRD DOG AND ROTATE

➡ 1 x 15 / side | p. 226

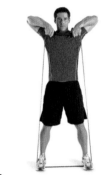

4
SB LATERAL WALK

➡ 1 x 15 / side | p. 243

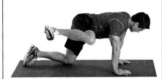

5
SB UPRIGHT ROW

➡ 1 x 15 | p. 243

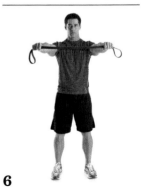

6
SB SPLITTER

➡ 1 x 15 | p. 242

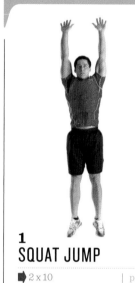

1
SQUAT JUMP
➡ 2 x 10 | p. 234

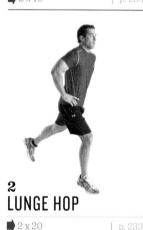

2
LUNGE HOP
➡ 2 x 20 | p. 233

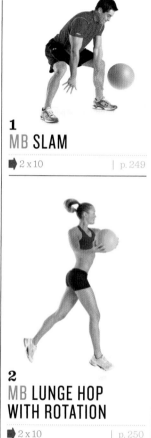

1
MB SLAM
➡ 2 x 10 | p. 249

2
MB LUNGE HOP WITH ROTATION
➡ 2 x 10 | p. 250

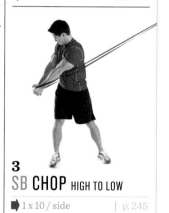

3
SB CHOP HIGH TO LOW
➡ 1 x 10 / side | p. 245

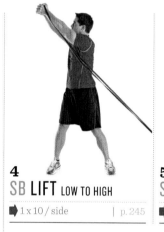

4
SB LIFT LOW TO HIGH
➡ 1 x 10 / side | p. 245

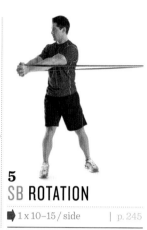

5
SB ROTATION
➡ 1 x 10–15 / side | p. 245

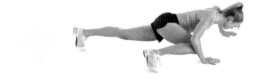

Upgrade the Dynamic Warmup /// During Stage II of the program, you'll slightly adjust the dynamic warmup. You'll still complete the 15 original exercises, but you'll also add a new movement: lizard crawls. This fun yet challenging movement combines a crawling motion with a pushup and will help prepare your upper body and core for your upcoming workout. Include lizard crawls as part of your warmup for the rest of the program.

WEEK 4
MON

IN SEASON

TOTAL-BODY WORKOUT

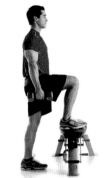

1a
KB SWING
➡ 3 x 15 | p. 251

2a
DB STEPUP
➡ 3 x 8–10 | p. 264

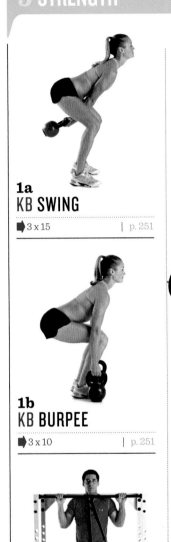

1b
KB BURPEE
➡ 3 x 10 | p. 251

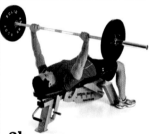

2b
BARBELL BENCH PRESS
➡ 3 x 15, 10, max | p. 266

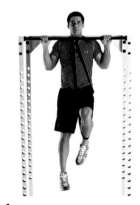

1c
SB PULLUP
➡ 3 x 5–10 | p. 246

2c
SB SQUAT AND SINGLE-ARM ROW AND ROTATE
➡ 3 x 10 / side | p. 247

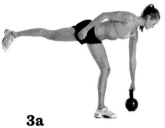

3a
KB SINGLE-LEG
ROMANIAN DEADLIFT
IPSILATERAL

➡ 2 x 12 | p. 252

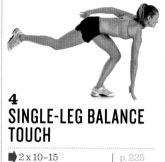

4
SINGLE-LEG BALANCE
TOUCH

➡ 2 x 10–15 | p. 225

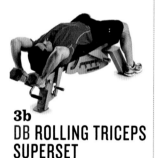

3b
DB ROLLING TRICEPS
SUPERSET

➡ 2 x 10 | p. 263

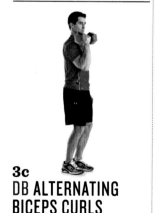

3c
DB ALTERNATING
BICEPS CURLS

➡ 2 x 10–15 | p. 258

GRAND FINALE
CONDITIONING
after workout

sprint 1	**1 MINUTE ON**
	1 MINUTE OFF
sprints 2–4	**30 SEC ON**
	30–60 SEC OFF
sprint 5	**Max duration**
	You choose speed

For each sprint, select a speed that is about 80% of your max so you can complete each set.

"The only way to discover the limits of the possible is to go beyond them into the impossible."

— ARTHUR C. CLARKE

WEEK 4 WED

IN SEASON

PLYOMETRICS & POWER
upper-body emphasis

1 THE DYNAMIC WARMUP

1 JUMPING JACK	7 LUNGE & ROTATE	12 SKIPPING BACKWARD
2 GATE SWING	8 REVERSE LUNGE & REACH OVER TOP	13 FRANKENSTEIN WALK
3 POGO HOP	9 CARIOCA	14 FRANKENSTEIN SKIP
4 SEAL JACK	10 LIZARD CRAWL	15 INCHWORM
5 BODYWEIGHT SQUAT	11 SKIPPING FORWARD	16 HIP SWING
6 SIDE LUNGE		

2 JOINT INTEGRITY

Rest approximately 30 seconds between exercises.

Shoulders

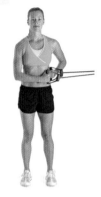
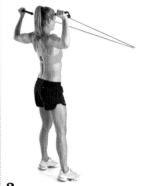

1
SC EXTERNAL ROTATION

➡ 1 x 15 / arm | p. 241

3
SC DOUBLE-ARM SCARECROW

➡ 1 x 15 | p. 242

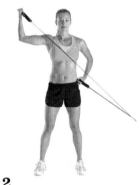
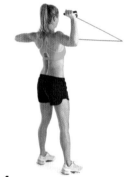

2
SC HITCHHIKER

➡ 1 x 15 / arm | p. 242

4
SC SINGLE-ARM SCARECROW

➡ 1 x max / arm | p. 241

3 PLYOMETRICS

Rest approximately
30 seconds between exercises.

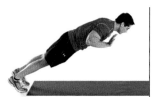

1
PLYO PUSHUP

➡ 2 x 10 | p. 229

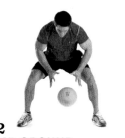

2
MB GROUND PUSH SLAM

➡ 2 x 10 | p. 249

4 CORE

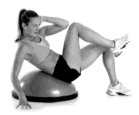

1
BOSU OPPOSITE ELBOW AND KNEE

➡ 1 x 15 / side | p. 240

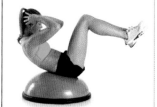

2
BOSU CRUNCH AND KICK

➡ 1 x 15 | p. 237

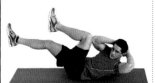

3
BICYCLE AND ROTATE

➡ 2 x max | p. 228

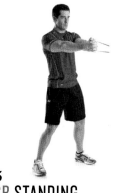

4
SB ROTATION

➡ 2 x 15 | p. 245

5
SB STANDING ANTIROTATION

➡ 1 x 15 / side | p. 244

IMPACT DICTIONARY

Split Fusion Workout

A training method consisting of 1 full-body training day per week and 2 training days that focus on the lower body 1 day and the upper body on the other day. This split will allow for increased volume and specific work to further accelerate your results. You'll still have your full-body training body-weight boot camp session as well.

4

WED

PLYOMETRICS & POWER
upper-body emphasis

5 STRENGTH

TRX UPPER-BODY BLAST

1a
TRX ROW
➡ 1 x 10–15 | p. 255

1b
TRX CHEST PRESS
➡ 1 x 10–15 | p. 256

1c
TRX TRICEPS EXTENSION
➡ 1 x 10–15 | p. 255

1d
TRX BICEPS CURL
➡ 1 x 10–15 | p. 257

1e
TRX I, Y, AND T DELTOID FLY
➡ 1 x 5 each | p. 256

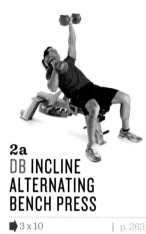

2a
DB INCLINE ALTERNATING BENCH PRESS

➡ 3 x 10 | p. 263

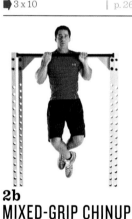

2b
MIXED-GRIP CHINUP

➡ 3 x 5–10 | p. 235

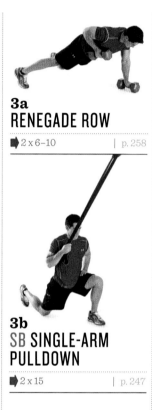

3a
RENEGADE ROW

➡ 2 x 6–10 | p. 258

3b
SB SINGLE-ARM PULLDOWN

➡ 2 x 15 | p. 247

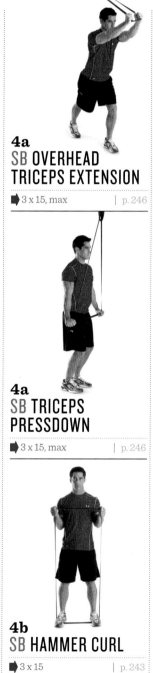

4a
SB OVERHEAD TRICEPS EXTENSION

➡ 3 x 15, max | p. 246

4a
SB TRICEPS PRESSDOWN

➡ 3 x 15, max | p. 246

4b
SB HAMMER CURL

➡ 3 x 15 | p. 243

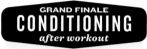

GRAND FINALE
CONDITIONING
after workout

Steady-state cardio
8–12 MINUTES
60–75% MHR

WEEK 4

THURS

PLYOMETRICS & POWER
upper-body emphasis

1 THE DYNAMIC WARMUP

1 JUMPING JACK	7 LUNGE & ROTATE	12 SKIPPING BACKWARD
2 GATE SWING	8 REVERSE LUNGE & REACH OVER TOP	13 FRANKENSTEIN WALK
3 POGO HOP	9 CARIOCA	14 FRANKENSTEIN SKIP
4 SEAL JACK	10 LIZARD CRAWL	15 INCHWORM
5 BODYWEIGHT SQUAT	11 SKIPPING FORWARD	16 HIP SWING
6 SIDE LUNGE		

2 JOINT INTEGRITY

Rest approximately 30 seconds between exercises.

Balance

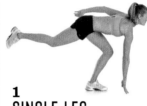

1
SINGLE-LEG BALANCE TOUCH

➡ 1 x 15 / leg | p. 225

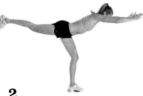

2
SINGLE-LEG BALANCE REACH-FORWARD

➡ 1 x 10 / leg | p. 230

GRAND FINALE
CONDITIONING
after workout

Sprinting
**20 SECONDS ON
30–45 SECONDS OFF**
5 sets
80-90% max effort

3 PLYOMETRICS

Complete all 3 exercises and then repeat circuit; 30 seconds between exercises; 1–2 minutes rest between circuits.

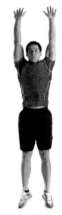

1
SQUAT JUMP

➡ 2 x 10 | p. 234

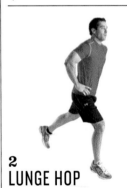

2
LUNGE HOP

➡ 2 x 20 | p. 233

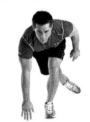

3
SKATER PLYO

➡ 2 x 20 | p. 230

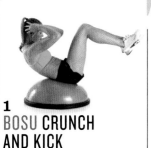

1
BOSU CRUNCH AND KICK

➡ 1 x 10 | p. 237

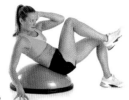

2
BOSU OPPOSITE ELBOW AND KNEE

➡ 2 x 15 / side | p. 240

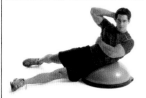

3
BOSU SIDEUP

➡ 1 x 15 / side | p. 237

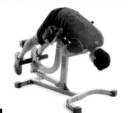

4
HYPEREXTENSION

➡ 2 x 10 | p. 234

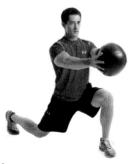

1a
MB DIAGONAL LUNGE WITH PRESS

➡ 3 x 20 | p. 249

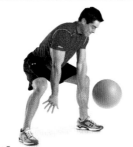

1b
MB SLAM

➡ 3 x 10 | p. 249

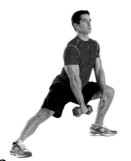

2a
DB SIDE LUNGE

➡ 2 x 10 / leg | p. 261

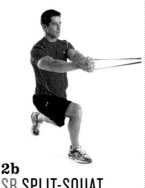

2b
SB SPLIT-SQUAT ANTIROTATION

➡ 1 x 10–15 / side | p. 244

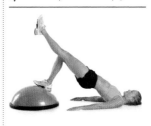

3a
BOSU SINGLE-LEG HIP BRIDGE

➡ 3 x 15 / leg | p. 238

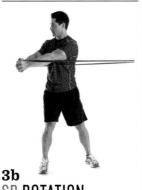

3b
SB ROTATION

➡ 3 x 10–15 / side | p. 245

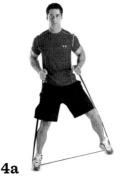

4a
SB LATERAL WALK

➡ 2 x 15 / side | p. 243

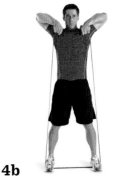

4b
SB UPRIGHT ROW

➡ 2 x 15 | p. 243

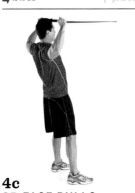

4c
SB FACE PULLS

➡ 2 x 15 | p. 243

WEEK 4 BOOT CAMP

1 TEN-MINUTE CARDIO

2 THE DYNAMIC WARMUP

1 JUMPING JACK	5 POGO HOP	8 CARIOCA
2 GATE SWING	6 REVERSE LUNGE/ ROTATION	9 FRANKENSTEIN WALK
3 PUSHUP	7 SKIPPING	10 INCHWORM
4 SEAL JACK		

CIRCUIT 1

Rest approximately 30 seconds between exercises.

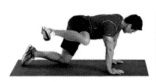

1
DIRTY DOG
➡ 1 x 15 / leg | p. 226

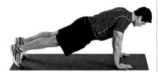

2
PUSHUP
➡ 1 x 15 | p. 229

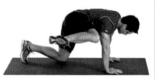

3
HORSEBACK RIDING
➡ 1 x 10 / leg | p. 227

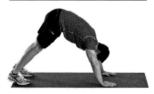

4
DIVEBOMBER PUSHUP
➡ 1 x 10 | p. 232

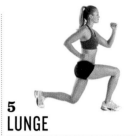

5
LUNGE
➡ 2 x 20 | p. 233

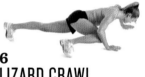

6
LIZARD CRAWL
➡ 2 x 10–20 | p. 224

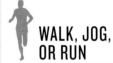

WALK, JOG, OR RUN
➡ 3–5 minutes

CIRCUIT 2

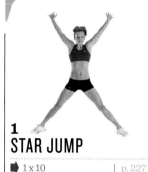

1
STAR JUMP
➡ 1 x 10 | p. 227

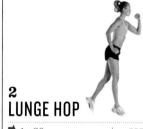

2
LUNGE HOP
➡ 1 x 20 | p. 233

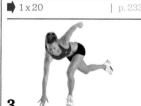

3
SKATER PLYO
➡ 1 x 20 | p. 230

4
SURFER
➡ 1 x 10 | p. 227

RUN
3–5 minutes

CIRCUIT 3

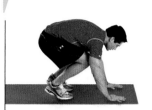

1
BURPEE
➡ 1 x 10 | p. 229

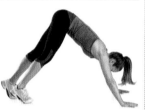

2
INCHWORM
➡ 1 x 10 | p. 224

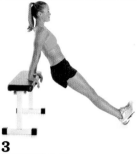

3
BENCH DIP
➡ 2 x 20 | p. 236

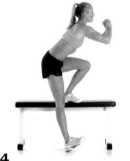

4
STEPDOWN
➡ 2 x 10–15 / leg | p. 236

RUN
➡ 3–5 minutes

GRAND FINALE
CONDITIONING
after workout

Sprint
**30 SECONDS ON
30–60 SECONDS OFF**
3–5 sets

CIRCUIT 4

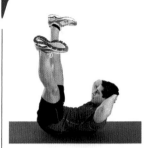

1
HELLO DOLLY
➡ 1 x 20 | p. 232

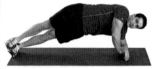

2
HIPUP
➡ 1 x 20 | p. 231

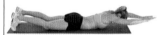

3
SWIMMER
➡ 1 x 15 | p. 230

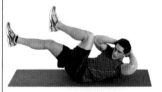

4
BICYCLE AND ROTATE
➡ 1 x max | p. 228

WEEK 5 MON

COMPLEX TRAINING
total-body workout

1 THE DYNAMIC WARMUP

1 JUMPING JACK	7 LUNGE & ROTATE	12 SKIPPING BACKWARD
2 GATE SWING	8 REVERSE LUNGE & REACH OVER TOP	13 FRANKENSTEIN WALK
3 POGO HOP	9 CARIOCA	14 FRANKENSTEIN SKIP
4 SEAL JACK	10 LIZARD CRAWL	15 WALKOUT
5 BODYWEIGHT SQUAT	11 SKIPPING FORWARD	16 HIP SWING
6 SIDE LUNGE		

2 JOINT INTEGRITY

Rest approximately 30 seconds between exercises.

Hips

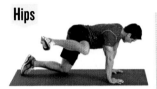

1
DIRTY DOG
➡ 2 x 15 / leg | p. 226

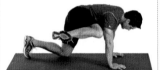

2
HORSEBACK RIDING
➡ 1 x 10 / leg | p. 227

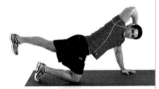

3
BIRD DOG AND ROTATE
➡ 1 x 15 / side | p. 226

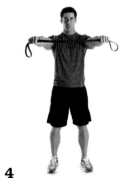

4
SB SPLITTER
➡ 1 x 15 | p. 242

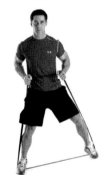

5
SB LATERAL WALK
➡ 1 x 15 / side | p. 243

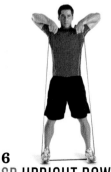

6
SB UPRIGHT ROW
➡ 1 x 15 | p. 243

3 CORE

Rest approximately 30 seconds between exercises.

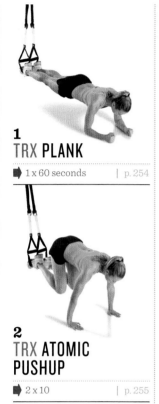

1
TRX PLANK

➡ 1 x 60 seconds | p. 254

2
TRX ATOMIC PUSHUP

➡ 2 x 10 | p. 255

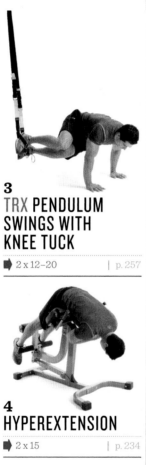

3
TRX PENDULUM SWINGS WITH KNEE TUCK

➡ 2 x 12–20 | p. 257

4
HYPEREXTENSION

➡ 2 x 15 | p. 234

4 STRENGTH

BUS DRIVER COMPLEX

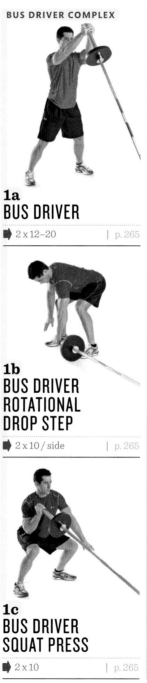

1a
BUS DRIVER

➡ 2 x 12–20 | p. 265

1b
BUS DRIVER ROTATIONAL DROP STEP

➡ 2 x 10 / side | p. 265

1c
BUS DRIVER SQUAT PRESS

➡ 2 x 10 | p. 265

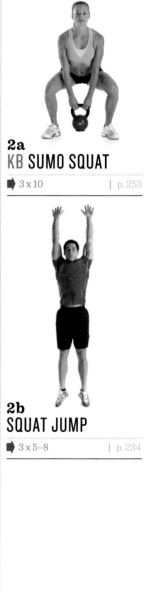

2a
KB SUMO SQUAT

➡ 3 x 10 | p. 253

2b
SQUAT JUMP

➡ 3 x 5–8 | p. 234

WEEK 5 MON

IN SEASON

COMPLEX TRAINING
total-body workout

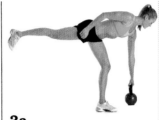

3a
KB SINGLE-LEG ROMANIAN DEADLIFT
IPSILATERAL

➡ 2 x 10 / leg | p. 252

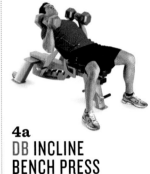

4a
DB INCLINE BENCH PRESS

➡ 3 x 15, 10, max | p. 263

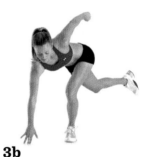

3b
SKATER PLYO

➡ 2 x 20 | p. 230

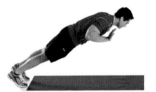

4b
PLYO PUSHUP

➡ 3 x 6–12 | p. 229

GRAND FINALE
CONDITIONING
after workout

sprint 1	**1 MINUTE ON** **1 MINUTE OFF**
sprint 2-5	**30 SEC ON** **30–60 SEC OFF**
sprint 6	**Max duration** You choose speed

*For each sprint, select a speed
that is about 80% of your max
so you can complete each set.*

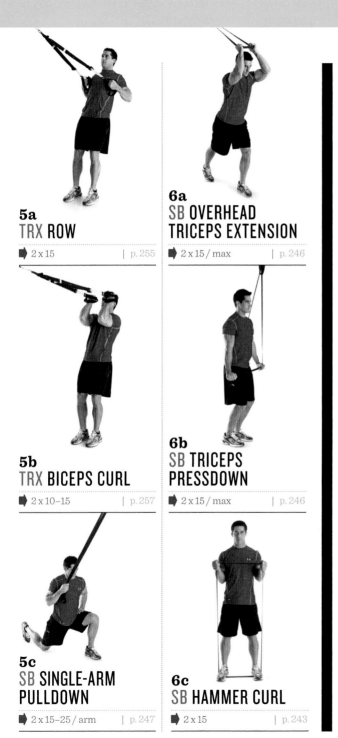

5a
TRX ROW

➡ 2 x 15 | p. 255

5b
TRX BICEPS CURL

➡ 2 x 10–15 | p. 257

5c
SB SINGLE-ARM PULLDOWN

➡ 2 x 15–25 / arm | p. 247

6a
SB OVERHEAD TRICEPS EXTENSION

➡ 2 x 15 / max | p. 246

6b
SB TRICEPS PRESSDOWN

➡ 2 x 15 / max | p. 246

6c
SB HAMMER CURL

➡ 2 x 15 | p. 243

IMPACT SECRETS *from the pros*

NICK HUNDLEY
CATCHER
SAN DIEGO PADRES

Todd Durkin client for 1 year

WHY HE NEEDS IMPACT TRAINING: "I had sports hernia surgery this past off-season, so I needed to rehabilitate my entire core, plus get the rest of my body in shape for Spring Training. That's a tall order."

WHEN HE REALIZED IMPACT MADE A DIFFERENCE: "The first day I did tractor tire flips in the parking lot and could feel in my core and lower body that I was all the way back from surgery. I knew I was where I needed to be and with whom I should be training."

HIS TRAINING SECRET: "Don't stop. If you never stop training, you don't lose your gains. I take as much of TD's workouts into the season as I can, training after games. It's the only way I'll stay in condition over the long haul of the season."

WEEK 5 WED

IN SEASON

COMPLEX TRAINING
upper-body emphasis

1 THE DYNAMIC WARMUP

1 JUMPING JACKS	7 LUNGE & ROTATE	12 SKIPPING BACKWARD
2 GATE SWING	8 REVERSE LUNGE & REACH OVER TOP	13 FRANKENSTEIN WALK
3 POGO HOP	9 CARIOCA	14 FRANKENSTEIN SKIP
4 SEAL JACK	10 LIZARD CRAWL	15 INCHWORM
5 BODY-WEIGHT SQUAT	11 SKIPPING FORWARD	16 HIP SWING
6 SIDE LUNGE		

2 JOINT INTEGRITY

Rest approximately 30 seconds between exercises.

Shoulders

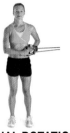

1
SC EXTERNAL ROTATION
➡ 2 x 15 / arm | p. 241

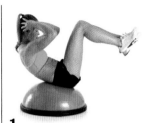

2
SC HITCHHIKER
➡ 2 x 15 / arm | p. 242

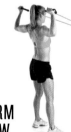

3
SC DOUBLE-ARM SCARECROW
➡ 2 x 15 | p. 242

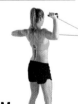

4
SC SINGLE-ARM SCARECROW
➡ 2 x 15 / arm | p. 241

3 CORE

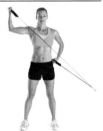

1
BOSU CRUNCH AND KICK
➡ 2 x 10 | p. 237

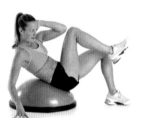

2
BOSU OPPOSITE ELBOW AND KNEE
➡ 2 x 15 | p. 240

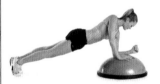

3
BOSU PLANK TO STAND
➡ 2 x 20 | p. 241

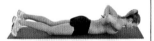

4
RUNNING-MAN SITUP
➡ 2 x 20 | p. 230

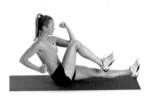

5
SWIMMER
➡ 2 x 15 | p. 230

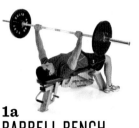

1a
BARBELL BENCH PRESS
➡ 3 x 15, 10, max | p. 266

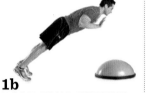

1b
BOSU PLYO PUSHUP
DOME UP
➡ 3 x 5–10 | p. 238

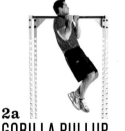

2a
GORILLA PULLUP
➡ 2 x max | p. 231

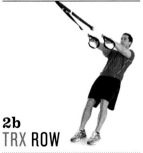

2b
TRX ROW
➡ 2 x 10–15 | p. 255

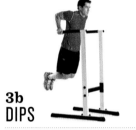

3a
DB INCLINE ALTERNATING BENCH PRESS
➡ 2 x 10 / arm | p. 263

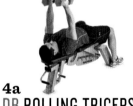

3b
DIPS
➡ 2 x 6–10 | p. 236

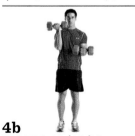

4a
DB ROLLING TRICEPS SUPERSET
➡ 2 x 10, 10–15 | p. 263

4b
BICEPS 10/10/10
➡ 2 sets | p. 262

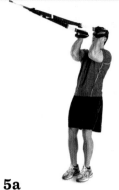

5a
TRX BICEPS CURL
➡ 2 x 10–15 | p. 257

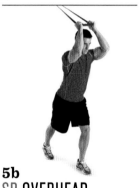

5b
SB OVERHEAD TRICEPS EXTENSION
➡ 2 x 10–15 | p. 246

GRAND FINALE
CONDITIONING
after workout

Steady-state cardio
8–12 MINUTES
60–75% MHR

WEEK 5 THURS

COMPLEX TRAINING
lower-body emphasis

1 THE DYNAMIC WARMUP

1 JUMPING JACK	7 LUNGE & ROTATE	12 SKIPPING BACKWARD
2 GATE SWING	8 REVERSE LUNGE & REACH OVER TOP	13 FRANKENSTEIN WALK
3 POGO HOP	9 CARIOCA	14 FRANKENSTEIN SKIP
4 SEAL JACK	10 LIZARD CRAWL	15 INCHWORM
5 BODYWEIGHT SQUAT	11 SKIPPING FORWARD	16 HIP SWING
6 SIDE LUNGE		

2 JOINT INTEGRITY

Rest approximately 30 seconds between exercises.

Balance

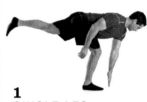

1 SINGLE-LEG ROTATIONAL TOUCH

➡ 1 x 15 / leg | p. 231

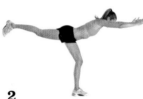

2 SINGLE-LEG BALANCE REACH-FORWARD

➡ 1 x 10 / side | p. 230

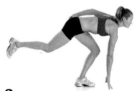

3 SINGLE-LEG BALANCE TOUCH AND HOP

➡ 1 x 10 / leg | p. 226

3 CORE

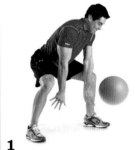

1 MB SLAM

➡ 2 x 10 | p. 249

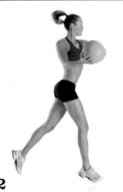

2 LUNGE HOP WITH MB ROTATION

➡ 2 x 10 | p. 250

GRAND FINALE
CONDITIONING
after workout

Sprint
80-90% max effort

**20 SECONDS ON
30-45 SECONDS OFF**

6 sets

Final sprint
1 MINUTE

Stride out and flush it out; approximately 50% of max effort.

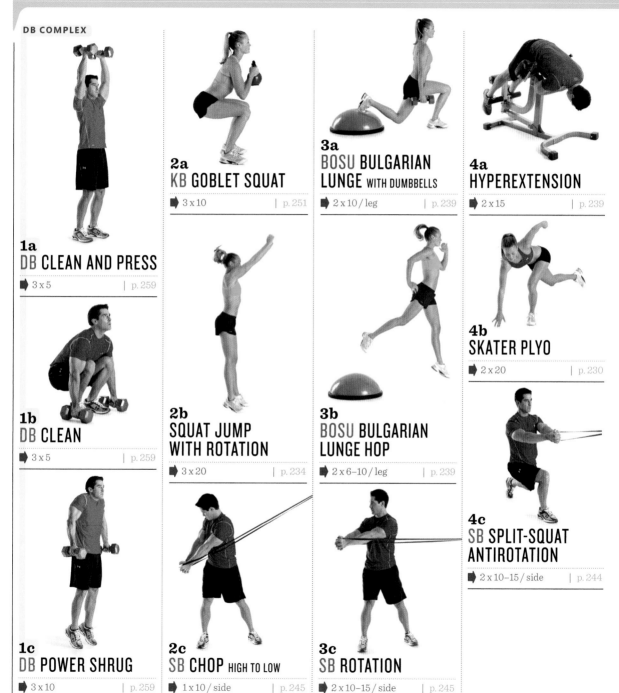

4 STRENGTH

DB COMPLEX

1a
DB CLEAN AND PRESS
➡ 3 x 5 | p. 259

1b
DB CLEAN
➡ 3 x 5 | p. 259

1c
DB POWER SHRUG
➡ 3 x 10 | p. 259

2a
KB GOBLET SQUAT
➡ 3 x 10 | p. 251

2b
SQUAT JUMP
WITH ROTATION
➡ 3 x 20 | p. 234

2c
SB CHOP HIGH TO LOW
➡ 1 x 10 / side | p. 245

3a
BOSU BULGARIAN
LUNGE WITH DUMBBELLS
➡ 2 x 10 / leg | p. 239

3b
BOSU BULGARIAN
LUNGE HOP
➡ 2 x 6–10 / leg | p. 239

3c
SB ROTATION
➡ 2 x 10–15 / side | p. 245

4a
HYPEREXTENSION
➡ 2 x 15 | p. 239

4b
SKATER PLYO
➡ 2 x 20 | p. 230

4c
SB SPLIT-SQUAT
ANTIROTATION
➡ 2 x 10–15 / side | p. 244

WEEK 5 BOOT CAMP

1 TEN-MINUTE CARDIO

2 THE DYNAMIC WARMUP

1 JUMPING JACK

2 GATE SWING

3 PUSHUP

4 SEAL JACK

5 POGO HOP

6 REVERSE LUNGE/ROTATION

7 SKIPPING

8 CARIOCA

9 FRANKENSTEIN WALK

10 INCHWORM

CIRCUIT 1

Rest approximately 30 seconds between exercises.

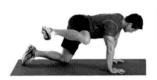

1 DIRTY DOG

➡ 1 x 15 / leg | p. 226

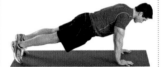

2 PUSHUP

➡ 1 x 15 | p. 229

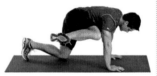

3 HORSEBACK RIDING

➡ 1 x 10 / leg | p. 227

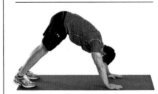

4 DIVEBOMBER PUSHUP

➡ 1 x 10 | p. 232

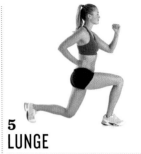

5 LUNGE

➡ 2 x 20 | p. 233

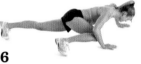

6 LIZARD CRAWL

➡ 2 x 10–20 | p. 224

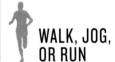

WALK, JOG, OR RUN

➡ 3–5 minutes

CIRCUIT 2

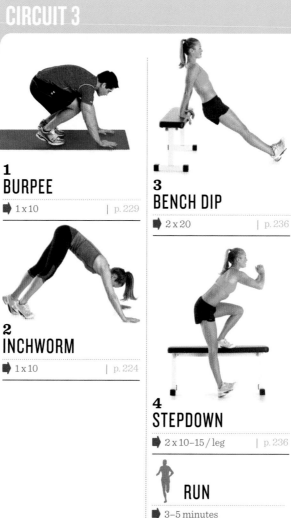

1
STAR JUMP
➡ 1 x 10 | p. 227

2
LUNGE HOP
➡ 1 x 20 | p. 233

3
SKATER PLYO
➡ 1 x 20 | p. 230

4
SURFER
➡ 1 x 10 | p. 227

RUN
➡ 3–5 minutes

CIRCUIT 3

1
BURPEE
➡ 1 x 10 | p. 229

2
INCHWORM
➡ 1 x 10 | p. 224

3
BENCH DIP
➡ 2 x 20 | p. 236

4
STEPDOWN
➡ 2 x 10–15 / leg | p. 236

RUN
➡ 3–5 minutes

GRAND FINALE
CONDITIONING
after workout

300-yard shuttle run
2-3 MINUTES OFF
Repeat 1 time

CIRCUIT 4

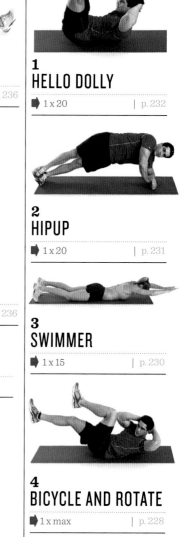

1
HELLO DOLLY
➡ 1 x 20 | p. 232

2
HIPUP
➡ 1 x 20 | p. 231

3
SWIMMER
➡ 1 x 15 | p. 230

4
BICYCLE AND ROTATE
➡ 1 x max | p. 228

WEEK 6 MON
IN SEASON

DROP SETS
total-body workout

1 THE DYNAMIC WARMUP

1 JUMPING JACK

2 GATE SWING

3 POGO HOP

4 SEAL JACK

5 BODYWEIGHT SQUAT

6 SIDE LUNGE

7 LUNGE & ROTATE

8 REVERSE LUNGE & REACH OVER TOP

9 CARIOCA

10 LIZARD CRAWL

11 SKIPPING FORWARD

12 SKIPPING BACKWARD

13 FRANKENSTEIN WALK

14 FRANKENSTEIN SKIP

15 INCHWORM

16 HIP SWING

2 JOINT INTEGRITY

Rest approximately 30 seconds between exercises.

Hips

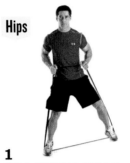

1
SB LATERAL WALK
➡ 2 x 15, max | p. 243

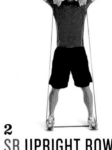

2
SB UPRIGHT ROW
➡ 2 x 15, max | p. 243

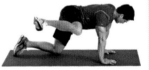

3
DIRTY DOG
➡ 2 x 15 / leg | p. 226

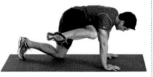

4
HORSEBACK RIDING
➡ 1 x 10 / leg | p. 227

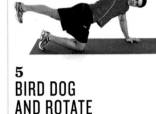

5
BIRD DOG AND ROTATE
➡ 1 x 15 / side | p. 226

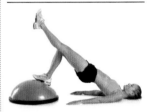

6
BOSU SINGLE-LEG HIP BRIDGE
➡ 2 x 15 / leg | p. 238

3 CORE

Rest approximately
30 seconds between exercises.

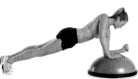

1
BOSU PLANK TO STAND

➡ 1 x 5–10 / arm | p. 241

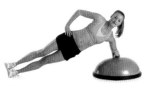

2
BOSU HIPUP

➡ 1 x 20 | p. 237

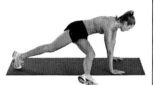

3
3-POINT CORE TUCK

➡ 2 x 15 | p. 232

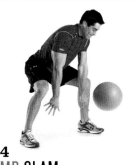

4
MB SLAM

➡ 2 x 10 | p. 249

4 STRENGTH

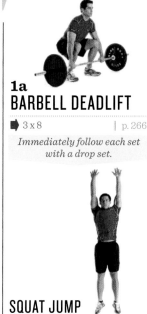

1a
BARBELL DEADLIFT

➡ 3 x 8 | p. 266

Immediately follow each set with a drop set.

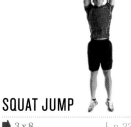

SQUAT JUMP

➡ 3 x 8 | p. 234

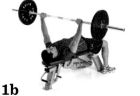

1b
BARBELL BENCH PRESS

➡ 3 x 10, 5, 5 | p. 266

Immediately follow each set with a drop set.

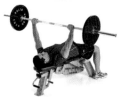

BARBELL BENCH PRESS

➡ 3 x 5–10 | p. 266

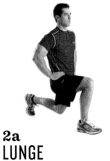

1c
PULLUP

➡ 3 x 5–10 | p. 235

Immediately follow each set with a drop set.

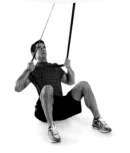

SB SEATED PULLDOWN

➡ 3 x 15 | p. 246

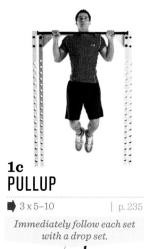

2a
LUNGE

➡ 2 x 20 | p. 233

Immediately follow each set with a drop set.

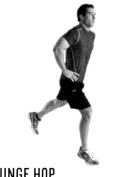

LUNGE HOP

➡ 2 x 20 | p. 233

IMPACT TIP

Drop set

A drop set consists of immediately following a regular set with another exercise using a weight that is 20 to 30 percent lighter.

WEEK 6 MON

IN SEASON

DROP SETS
total-body workout

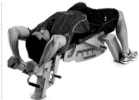

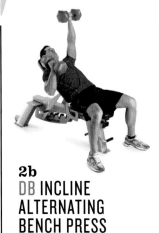

2b
DB INCLINE ALTERNATING BENCH PRESS

➡ 2 x 5 / arm | p. 263

Immediately follow each set with a drop set.

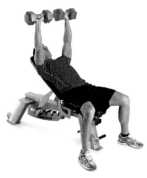

DB INCLINE BENCH PRESS

➡ 2 x 10 | p. 263

2c
DB ROLLING TRICEPS SUPERSET

➡ 3 x 5–10 | p. 263

Immediately followed by

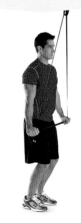

SB PRESSDOWN

➡ 3 x max | p. 246

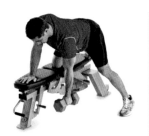

3a
DB SINGLE-ARM ROW

➡ 2 x 10 / arm | p. 261

Immediately followed by

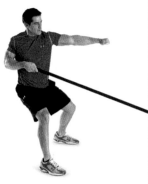

SB SQUAT AND SINGLE-ARM ROW AND ROTATE

➡ 2 x 10 / arm | p. 247

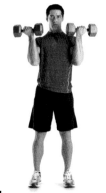

3b
DB BICEPS CURL

➡ 2 x 8 / arm | p. 257

Immediately follow each set with a drop set.

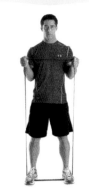

SB HAMMER CURL

➡ 2 x 10–15 | p. 243

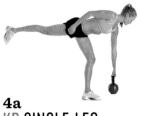

4a
KB SINGLE-LEG ROMANIAN DEADLIFT
IPSILATERAL

➡ 2 x 8 / leg | p. 252

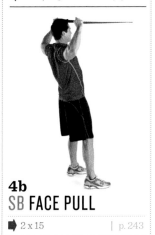

4b
SB FACE PULL

➡ 2 x 15 | p. 243

GRAND FINALE
CONDITIONING
after workout

sprint 1	**1 MINUTE ON 1 MINUTE OFF**
sprints 2–5	**30 SEC ON 30–60 SEC OFF**
sprint 6	**Max duration** You choose speed

For each sprint, select a speed that is about 80% of your max so you can complete each set.

WEEK 6

WED

IN SEASON

DROP SETS
upper-body emphasis

1 THE DYNAMIC WARMUP

1 JUMPING JACK	7 LUNGE & ROTATE	12 SKIPPING BACKWARD
2 GATE SWING	8 REVERSE LUNGE & REACH OVER TOP	13 FRANKENSTEIN WALK
3 POGO HOP	9 CARIOCA	14 FRANKENSTEIN SKIP
4 SEAL JACK	10 LIZARD CRAWL	15 INCHWORM
5 BODYWEIGHT SQUAT	11 SKIPPING FORWARD	16 HIP SWING
6 SIDE LUNGE		

2 JOINT INTEGRITY

Rest approximately 30 seconds between exercises.

Shoulders

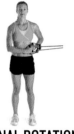

1
SC EXTERNAL ROTATION
2 x 15 / arm | p. 241

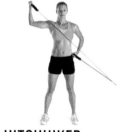

2
SC HITCHHIKER
2 x 15 / arm | p. 242

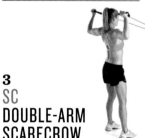

3
SC DOUBLE-ARM SCARECROW
2 x 15 | p. 242

4
SC SINGLE-ARM SCARECROW
2 x 15 / arm | p. 241

3 CORE

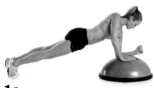

1a
BOSU PLANK TO STAND
1 x 5–10 | p. 241

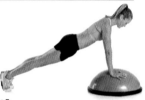

1b
BOSU PUSHUP
1 x 10 | p. 239

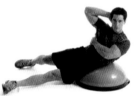

2a
BOSU SIDEUP
1 x 20 / side | p. 237

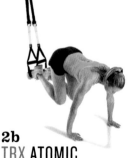

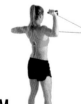

2b
TRX ATOMIC PUSHUP
2 x 10–15 | p. 255

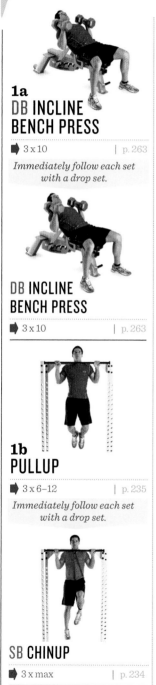

1a
DB INCLINE
BENCH PRESS

➡ 3 x 10 | p. 263

*Immediately follow each set
with a drop set.*

DB INCLINE
BENCH PRESS

➡ 3 x 10 | p. 263

1b
PULLUP

➡ 3 x 6–12 | p. 235

*Immediately follow each set
with a drop set.*

SB CHINUP

➡ 3 x max | p. 234

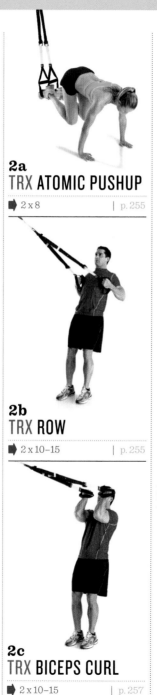

2a
TRX ATOMIC PUSHUP

➡ 2 x 8 | p. 255

2b
TRX ROW

➡ 2 x 10–15 | p. 255

2c
TRX BICEPS CURL

➡ 2 x 10–15 | p. 257

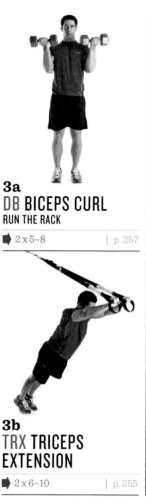

3a
DB BICEPS CURL
RUN THE RACK

➡ 2 x 5–8 | p. 257

3b
TRX TRICEPS
EXTENSION

➡ 2 x 6–10 | p. 255

IMPACT DICTIONARY

Run the Rack

A training method
consisting of 1 full-
body training day per
week and 2 training
days that focus on the
lower body 1 day and
the upper body on the
other day. This split
will allow for increased
volume and specific
work to further acceler-
ate your results. You'll
still have your full-body
training bodyweight
boot camp session
as well.

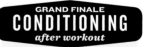

GRAND FINALE
CONDITIONING
after workout

Steady-state cardio
8-12 MINUTES
60–75% MHR

WEEK 6

THURS

DROP SETS
lower-body emphasis

1 THE DYNAMIC WARMUP

1 JUMPING JACK	7 LUNGE & ROTATE	12 SKIPPING BACKWARD
2 GATE SWING	8 REVERSE LUNGE & REACH OVER TOP	13 FRANKENSTEIN WALK
3 POGO HOP	9 CARIOCA	14 FRANKENSTEIN SKIP
4 SEAL JACK	10 LIZARD CRAWL	15 INCHWORM
5 BODYWEIGHT SQUAT	11 SKIPPING FORWARD	16 HIP SWING
6 SIDE LUNGE		

2 JOINT INTEGRITY

Rest approximately
30 seconds between exercises.

Balance

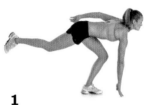

1
SINGLE-LEG BALANCE TOUCH
➡ 1 x 15 / leg | p. 225

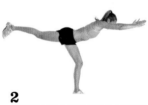

2
SINGLE-LEG BALANCE REACH-FORWARD
➡ 1 x 10 / leg | p. 230

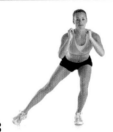

3
3-POINT BALANCE TOUCH
➡ 1 x 10 / leg | p. 225

3 CORE

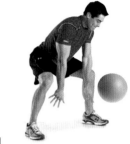

1
MB SLAM
➡ 2 x 10 | p. 249

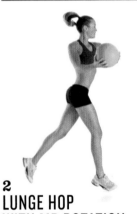

2
LUNGE HOP WITH MB ROTATION
➡ 2 x 20 | p. 250

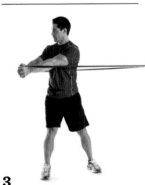

3
SB ROTATION
➡ 2 x 10–15 / side | p. 245

DB COMPLEX

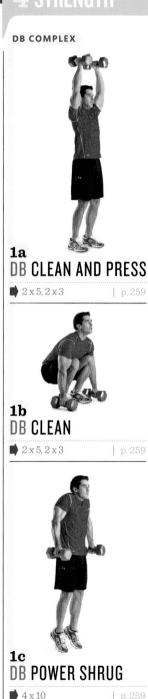

1a
DB CLEAN AND PRESS
➡ 2 x 5, 2 x 3 | p. 259

1b
DB CLEAN
➡ 2 x 5, 2 x 3 | p. 259

1c
DB POWER SHRUG
➡ 4 x 10 | p. 259

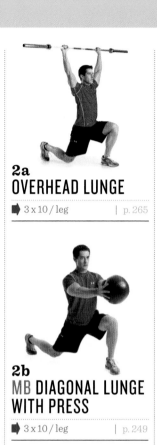

2a
OVERHEAD LUNGE
➡ 3 x 10 / leg | p. 265

2b
MB DIAGONAL LUNGE WITH PRESS
➡ 3 x 10 / leg | p. 249

2c
BOSU OPPOSITE ELBOW AND KNEE
➡ 3 x 15 / side | p. 240

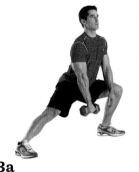

3a
DB SIDE LUNGE
➡ 2 x 10 / side | p. 261

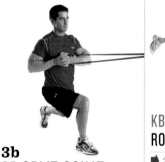

3b
SB SPLIT-SQUAT ANTIROTATION
➡ 2 x 10 / side | p. 244

GRAND FINALE
CONDITIONING
after workout

Sprinting
80-90% max effort

**20–30 SECONDS ON
30–45 SECONDS OFF**

6 sets

Final sprint
1 MINUTE

*Stride out and flush it out;
approximately 50% of max effort*

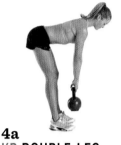

4a
KB DOUBLE-LEG ROMANIAN DEADLIFT
➡ 2 x 15 | p. 252

*Immediately follow each set
with a drop set.*

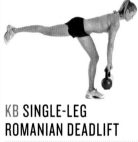

KB SINGLE-LEG ROMANIAN DEADLIFT
➡ 2 x 8 / leg | p. 252

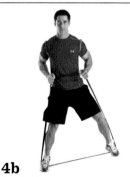

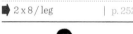

4b
SB LATERAL WALK
➡ 2 x 15 | p. 243

WEEK 6 BOOT CAMP

1 TEN-MINUTE CARDIO

2 THE DYNAMIC WARMUP

1 JUMPING JACK
2 GATE SWING
3 PUSHUP
4 SEAL JACK

5 POGO HOP
6 REVERSE LUNGE & REACH OVER TOP
7 SKIPPING

8 CARIOCA
9 FRANKENSTEIN WALK
10 INCHWORM

CIRCUIT I

Rest approximately 30 seconds between exercises.

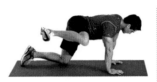

1 DIRTY DOG
➡ 1 x 15 / leg | p. 226

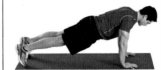

2 PUSHUP
➡ 1 x 15 | p. 229

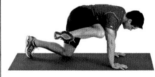

3 HORSEBACK RIDING
➡ 1 x 10 / leg | p. 227

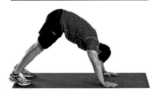

4 DIVEBOMBER PUSHUP
➡ 1 x 10 | p. 232

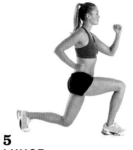

5 LUNGE
➡ 2 x 20 | p. 233

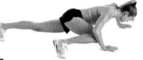

6 LIZARD CRAWL
➡ 2 x 10–20 | p. 224

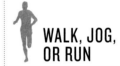

WALK, JOG, OR RUN
➡ 3–5 minutes

CIRCUIT 2

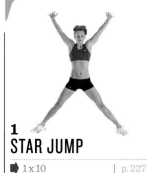

1
STAR JUMP
➡ 1 x 10 | p. 227

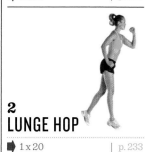

2
LUNGE HOP
➡ 1 x 20 | p. 233

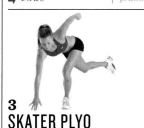

3
SKATER PLYO
➡ 1 x 20 | p. 230

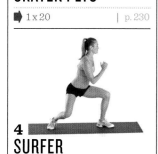

4
SURFER
➡ 1 x 10 | p. 227

RUN
➡ 3–5 minutes

CIRCUIT 3

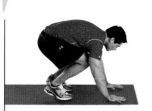

1
BURPEE
➡ 1 x 10 | p. 229

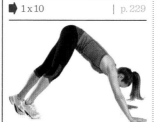

2
INCHWORM
➡ 1 x 10 | p. 224

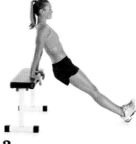

3
BENCH DIP
➡ 1 x 20 | p. 236

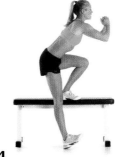

4
STEPDOWN
➡ 2 x 10–15 / leg | p. 236

RUN
➡ 3–5 minutes

GRAND FINALE
CONDITIONING
after workout

300-yard shuttle run
2–3 MINUTES OFF
Repeat 1 time

CIRCUIT 4

1
HELLO DOLLY
➡ 1 x 20 | p. 232

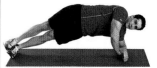

2
HIPUP
➡ 1 x 20 | p. 231

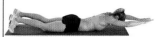

3
SWIMMER
➡ 1 x 15 | p. 230

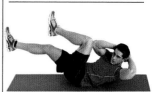

4
BICYCLE AND ROTATE
➡ 1 x max | p. 228

WEEK 7

MON

ECCENTRIC TRAINING
total-body workout

1 THE DYNAMIC WARMUP

1 JUMPING JACK	7 LUNGE & ROTATE	12 SKIPPING BACKWARD
2 GATE SWING	8 REVERSE LUNGE & REACH OVER TOP	13 FRANKENSTEIN WALK
3 POGO HOP	9 CARIOCA	14 FRANKENSTEIN SKIP
4 SEAL JACK	10 LIZARD CRAWL	15 INCHWORM
5 BODYWEIGHT SQUAT	11 SKIPPING FORWARD	16 HIP SWING
6 SIDE LUNGE		

2 JOINT INTEGRITY

Hips

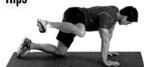

1
DIRTY DOG

➡ 2 x 15 / leg | p. 226

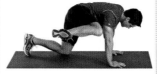

2
HORSEBACK RIDING

➡ 1 x 10 / leg | p. 227

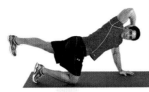

3
BIRD DOG AND ROTATE

➡ 1 x 15 / side | p. 226

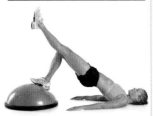

4
BOSU SINGLE-LEG HIP BRIDGE

➡ 2 x 15 / leg | p. 238

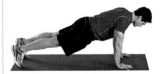

5
PUSHUP ECCENTRIC

➡ 2 x 10 | p. 229

3 POWER

Rest approximately 30 seconds between exercises.

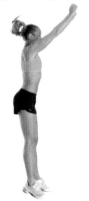

1
SQUAT JUMP WITH ROTATION

➡ 2 x 10 | p. 234

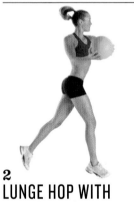

2
LUNGE HOP WITH MB ROTATION

➡ 2 x 20 | p. 250

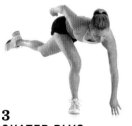

3
SKATER PLYO

➡ 2 x 20 | p. 230

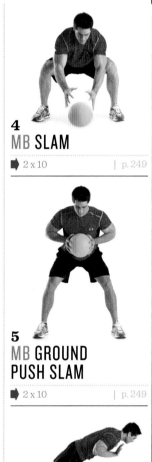

4
MB SLAM

➡ 2 x 10 | p. 249

5
MB GROUND PUSH SLAM

➡ 2 x 10 | p. 249

6
PLYO PUSHUP

➡ 2 x 10 | p. 229

4 CORE

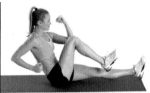

1
RUNNING-MAN SITUP

➡ 2 x 20 | p. 230

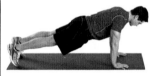

2
STANDING PLANK

➡ 1 x 30–60 seconds | p. 228

BUS DRIVER COMPLEX

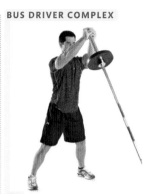

3a
BUS DRIVER

➡ 1 x 12–20 | p. 265

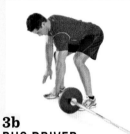

3b
BUS DRIVER ROTATIONAL DROP STEP

➡ 1 x 10 / side | p. 265

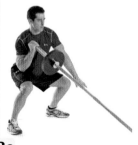

3c
BUS DRIVER SQUAT PRESS

➡ 1 x 10 / arm | p. 265

WEEK 7 MON

ECCENTRIC TRAINING
total-body workout

GRAND FINALE
CONDITIONING
after workout

sprint 1	**1 MINUTE ON** **1 MINUTE OFF**
sprints 2–5	**30 SEC ON** **30–60 SEC OFF**
sprint 6	**Max duration** You choose speed

For each sprint, select a speed that is about 80% of your max so you can complete each set.

5 STRENGTH

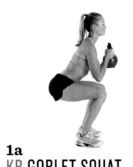

1a
KB GOBLET SQUAT
➡ 3 x 10 | p. 251

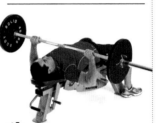

1b
BARBELL BENCH PRESS ECCENTRIC
➡ 3 x 5–8 | p. 266

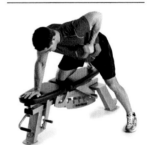

1c DB SINGLE-ARM ROW
➡ 3 x 10 / arm | p. 261

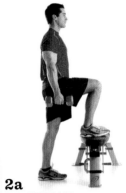

2a
DB STEPUP
➡ 3 x 8 / leg | p. 264

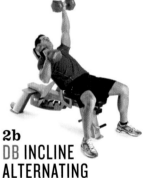

2b
DB INCLINE ALTERNATING BENCH PRESS
➡ 3 x 12, 8–10, 5–8 | p. 263

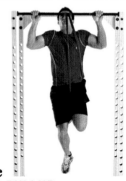

2c
SB PULLUP ECCENTRIC
➡ 3 x 5–8 | p. 246

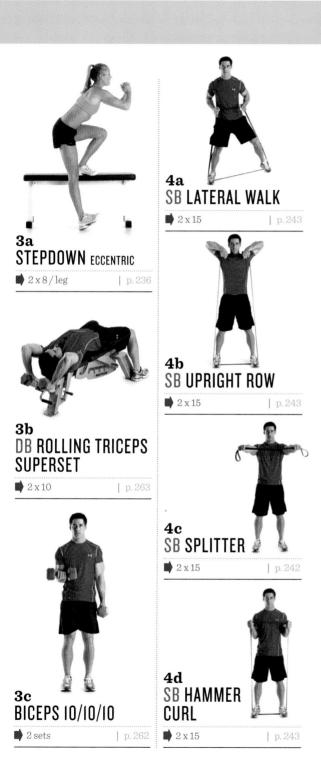

3a
STEPDOWN ECCENTRIC
➡ 2 x 8 / leg | p. 236

3b
DB ROLLING TRICEPS SUPERSET
➡ 2 x 10 | p. 263

3c
BICEPS 10/10/10
➡ 2 sets | p. 262

4a
SB LATERAL WALK
➡ 2 x 15 | p. 243

4b
SB UPRIGHT ROW
➡ 2 x 15 | p. 243

4c
SB SPLITTER
➡ 2 x 15 | p. 242

4d
SB HAMMER CURL
➡ 2 x 15 | p. 243

IMPACT DICTIONARY

Eccentric Training

In Week 7, you'll be introduced to eccentric training. This technique has commonly been referred to as "negatives" because you lower the weight slowly during the negative—or lowering—portion of the movement. I've decided not to use the term negative, because there is nothing negative about this very positive type of training. We'll call it by its scientific name: eccentric training.

When doing eccentric training, you have approximately 120 percent of the strength on the eccentric (lowering) phase that you have in the lifting phase because your muscles can oppose more force than they can generate. It's easier to lower a weight slowly during a bench press (you are resisting or opposing the force of the weight) than it is to press it up off your chest quickly (generating power by pushing).

Besides allowing you to use more weight, focusing on the eccentric portion of an exercise actually leads to more muscle growth. That's because your muscles elongate during the eccentric portion of the exercise, which causes more muscle recruitment. You should take 4 to 6 seconds to lower the weight (slower than gravity), depending on the movement, and have a spotter assist you back to the starting position. You will typically decrease your reps and increase the weight when performing eccentric reps. Eccentric training is a great way to overcome plateaus and increase your overall strength.

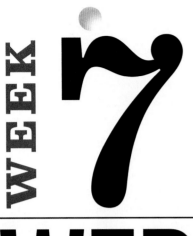

WEEK 7

WED

IN SEASON

ECCENTRIC TRAINING
upper-body emphasis

1 THE DYNAMIC WARMUP

1 JUMPING JACK	7 LUNGE & ROTATE	12 SKIPPING BACKWARD
2 GATE SWING	8 REVERSE LUNGE & REACH OVER TOP	13 FRANKENSTEIN WALK
3 POGO HOP	9 CARIOCA	14 FRANKENSTEIN SKIP
4 SEAL JACK	10 LIZARD CRAWL	15 INCHWORM
5 BODYWEIGHT SQUAT	11 SKIPPING FORWARD	16 HIP SWING
6 SIDE LUNGE		

2 JOINT INTEGRITY

Rest approximately
30 seconds between exercises.

Shoulders

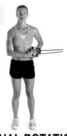

1
SC EXTERNAL ROTATION

➡ 2 x 15 / arm | p. 241

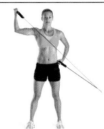

2
SC HITCHHIKER

➡ 2 x 15 / arm | p. 242

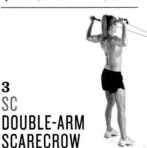

3
SC
DOUBLE-ARM
SCARECROW

➡ 2 x 15 | p. 242

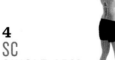

4
SC
SINGLE-ARM
SCARECROW

➡ 2 x 15 / arm

3 CORE

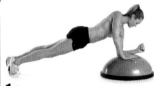

1a
BOSU PLANK TO
STAND

➡ 2 x 5–10 / side | p. 241

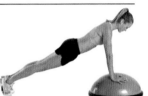

1b
BOSU PUSHUP
ECCENTRIC

➡ 1 x 6–10 | p. 239

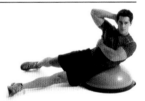

2a
BOSU SIDEUP

➡ 1 x 20 / side | p. 237

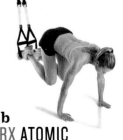

2b
TRX ATOMIC
PUSHUP

➡ 2 x 10–15 | p. 255

1a
BARBELL BENCH
PRESS ECCENTRIC
➡ 1 x 10, 3 x 5 | p. 266

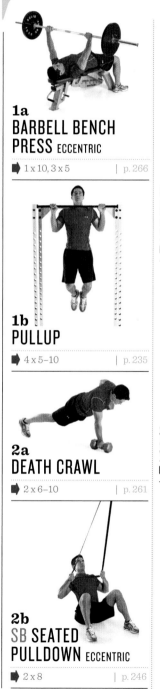

1b
PULLUP
➡ 4 x 5–10 | p. 235

2a
DEATH CRAWL
➡ 2 x 6–10 | p. 261

2b
SB SEATED
PULLDOWN ECCENTRIC
➡ 2 x 8 | p. 246

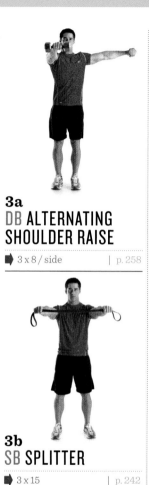

3a
DB ALTERNATING
SHOULDER RAISE
➡ 3 x 8 / side | p. 258

3b
SB SPLITTER
➡ 3 x 15 | p. 242

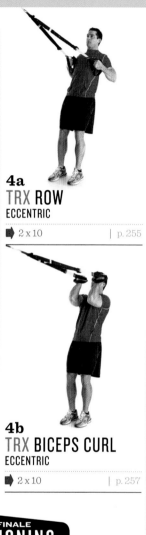

4a
TRX ROW
ECCENTRIC
➡ 2 x 10 | p. 255

4b
TRX BICEPS CURL
ECCENTRIC
➡ 2 x 10 | p. 257

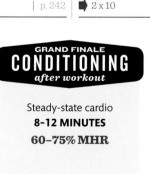

GRAND FINALE
CONDITIONING
after workout

Steady-state cardio
8-12 MINUTES
60-75% MHR

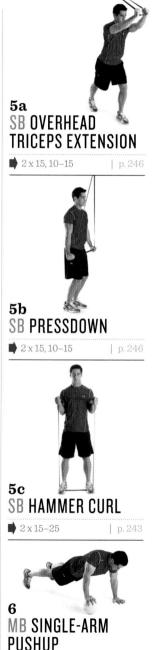

5a
SB OVERHEAD
TRICEPS EXTENSION
➡ 2 x 15, 10–15 | p. 246

5b
SB PRESSDOWN
➡ 2 x 15, 10–15 | p. 246

5c
SB HAMMER CURL
➡ 2 x 15–25 | p. 243

6
MB SINGLE-ARM
PUSHUP
➡ 2 x max | p. 248

WEEK 7 THURS

ECCENTRIC TRAINING
lower-body emphasis

1 THE DYNAMIC WARMUP

1 JUMPING JACK

2 GATE SWING

3 POGO HOP

4 SEAL JACK

5 BODYWEIGHT SQUAT

6 SIDE LUNGE

7 LUNGE & ROTATE

8 REVERSE LUNGE & REACH OVER TOP

9 CARIOCA

10 LIZARD CRAWL

11 SKIPPING FORWARD

12 SKIPPING BACKWARD

13 FRANKENSTEIN WALK

14 FRANKENSTEIN SKIP

15 INCHWORM

16 HIP SWING

2 JOINT INTEGRITY

Hips

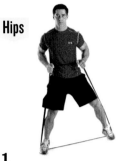

1 SB LATERAL WALK
➡ 2 x 15 | p. 243

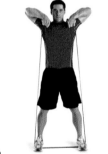

2 SB UPRIGHT ROW
➡ 2 x 15 | p. 243

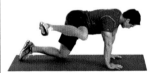

3 DIRTY DOG
➡ 2 x 15 / leg | p. 226

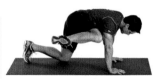

4 HORSEBACK RIDING
➡ 1 x 10 / leg | p. 227

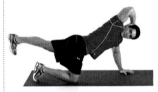

5 BIRD DOG AND ROTATE
➡ 1 x 15 / side | p. 226

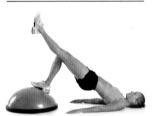

6 BOSU SINGLE-LEG HIP BRIDGE
➡ 2 x 15 | p. 238

3 PLYOS

Rest approximately 30 seconds between exercises. Repeat circuit.

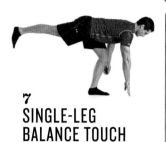

7
SINGLE-LEG BALANCE TOUCH

➡ 1 x 15 / leg | p. 225

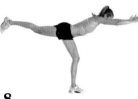

8
SINGLE-LEG BALANCE REACH-FORWARD

➡ 1 x 10 / leg | p. 230

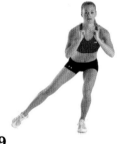

9
3-POINT BALANCE TOUCH

➡ 1 x 10 / leg | p. 225

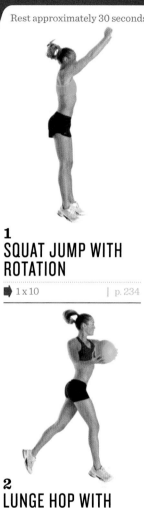

1
SQUAT JUMP WITH ROTATION

➡ 1 x 10 | p. 234

2
LUNGE HOP WITH MB ROTATION

➡ 1 x 20 | p. 250

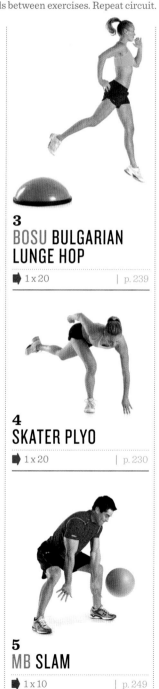

3
BOSU BULGARIAN LUNGE HOP

➡ 1 x 20 | p. 239

4
SKATER PLYO

➡ 1 x 20 | p. 230

5
MB SLAM

➡ 1 x 10 | p. 249

WEEK 7

THURS

ECCENTRIC TRAINING
lower-body emphasis

DB COMPLEX

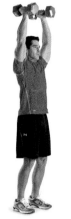

1a
DB CLEAN AND PRESS
➡ 2 x 5, 2 x 3 | p. 259

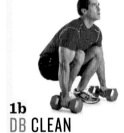

1b
DB CLEAN
➡ 2 x 5, 2 x 3 | p. 259

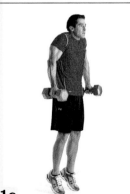
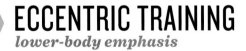

1c
DB POWER SHRUG
➡ 4 x 10 | p. 259

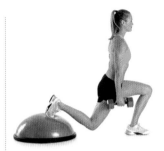

2a
BOSU BULGARIAN LUNGE ECCENTRIC
➡ 2 x 8 / leg | p. 239

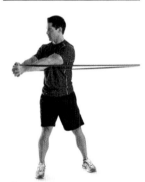

2b
SB ROTATION
➡ 2 x 15 / side | p. 245

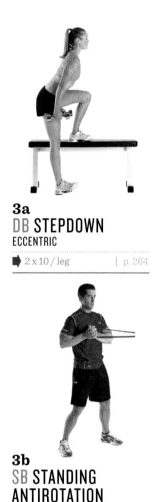

3a
DB STEPDOWN
ECCENTRIC

➡ 2 x 10 / leg | p. 264

3b
SB STANDING
ANTIROTATION

➡ 2 x 10 | p. 244

*"**When you change
the way you
look at things,
the things
you look at change.**"*

— DR. WAYNE DYER

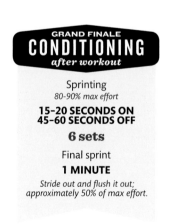

GRAND FINALE
CONDITIONING
after workout

Sprinting
80-90% max effort

15–20 SECONDS ON
45–60 SECONDS OFF

6 sets

Final sprint
1 MINUTE

Stride out and flush it out;
approximately 50% of max effort.

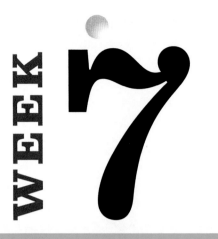

WEEK 7
BOOT CAMP

1 TEN-MINUTE CARDIO

2 THE DYNAMIC WARMUP

1 JUMPING JACK	5 POGO HOP	8 CARIOCA
2 GATE SWING	6 REVERSE LUNGE & REACH OVER TOP	9 FRANKENSTEIN WALK
3 PUSHUP	7 SKIPPING	10 INCHWORM
4 SEAL JACK		

CIRCUIT I

Rest approximately 30 seconds between exercises.

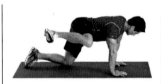

1
DIRTY DOG
➡ 1 x 15 / leg | p. 226

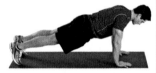

2
PUSHUP
➡ 1 x 15 | p. 229

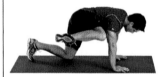

3
HORSEBACK RIDING
➡ 1 x 10 / leg | p. 227

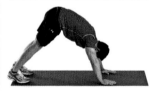

4
DIVEBOMBER PUSHUP
➡ 1 x 10 | p. 232

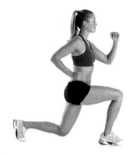

5
LUNGE
➡ 1 x 20 | p. 233

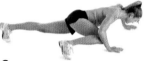

6
LIZARD CRAWL
➡ 1 x 10–20 | p. 224

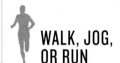

WALK, JOG, OR RUN
➡ 3–5 minutes

CIRCUIT 2

Complete circuit 2 times,
and then run.

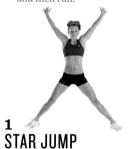

1
STAR JUMP

1 x 10 | p. 227

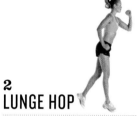

2
LUNGE HOP

1 x 20 | p. 233

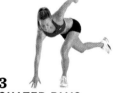

3
SKATER PLYO

1 x 20 | p. 230

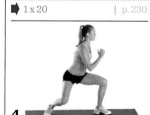

4
SURFER

1 x 10 | p. 227

RUN

3–5 minutes

CIRCUIT 3

Complete circuit 2 times, and then run.

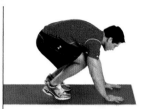

1
BURPEE

1 x 10 | p. 229

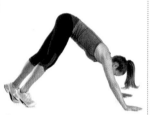

2
INCHWORM

1 x 10 | p. 224

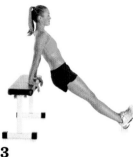

3
BENCH DIP

1 x 20 | p. 236

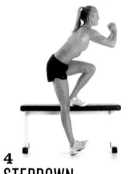

4
STEPDOWN

1 x 10–15 / leg | p. 236

RUN

3–5 minutes

GRAND FINALE
CONDITIONING
after workout

Sprint
**30 SECONDS ON
30–60 SECONDS OFF**
3 sets

CIRCUIT 4

Complete circuit 2 times.

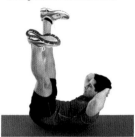

1
HELLO DOLLY

1 x 20 | p. 232

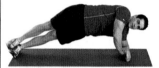

2
HIPUP

1 x 20 | p. 231

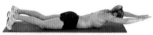

3
SWIMMER

1 x 15 | p. 230

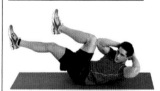

4
BICYCLE AND ROTATE

1 x max | p. 228

WEEK 8 MON

THE PLAYOFFS

MASTERING THE MATRIX
total-body workout

1 THE DYNAMIC WARMUP

1 JUMPING JACK	7 LUNGE & ROTATE	12 SKIPPING BACKWARD
2 GATE SWING	8 REVERSE LUNGE & REACH OVER TOP	13 FRANKENSTEIN WALK
3 POGO HOP	9 CARIOCA	14 FRANKENSTEIN SKIP
4 SEAL JACK	10 LIZARD CRAWL	15 INCHWORM
5 BODYWEIGHT SQUAT	11 SKIPPING FORWARD	16 HIP SWING
6 SIDE LUNGE		

2 JOINT INTEGRITY

Rest approximately
30 seconds between exercises.

Hips

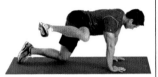

1
DIRTY DOG
➡ 2 x 15 / leg | p. 226

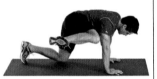

2
HORSEBACK RIDING
➡ 2 x 10 / leg | p. 227

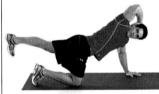

3
BIRD DOG AND ROTATE
➡ 2 x 15 / side | p. 226

3 POWER

Complete as a circuit, repeating
once. Rest approximately
30 seconds between exercises.

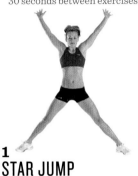

1
STAR JUMP
➡ 1 x 10 | p. 227

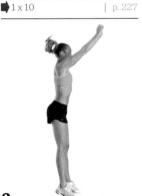

2
SQUAT JUMP WITH ROTATION
➡ 1 x 8 | p. 234

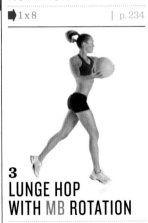

3
LUNGE HOP WITH MB ROTATION
➡ 1 x 20 | p. 250

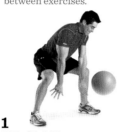

4 SKATER PLYO
➡ 1 x 20 | p. 230

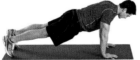

5 BOSU BULGARIAN LUNGE HOP
➡ 1 x 10–15 / leg | p. 239

4 CORE

Complete as a circuit. Rest about 30 seconds between exercises.

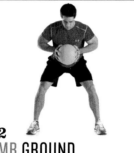

1 MB SLAM
➡ 2 x 10 | p. 249

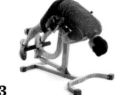

2 MB GROUND PUSH SLAM
➡ 2 x 10 | p. 249

3 HYPEREXTENSION
➡ 2 x 10–15 | p. 234

4 PUSHUP ECCENTRIC
➡ 2 x 5 | p. 229

5 STRENGTH

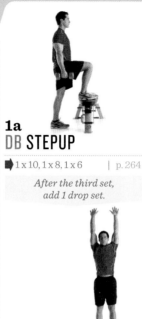

1a DB STEPUP
➡ 1 x 10, 1 x 8, 1 x 6 | p. 264

After the third set, add 1 drop set.

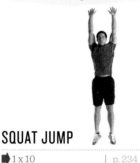

SQUAT JUMP
➡ 1 x 10 | p. 234

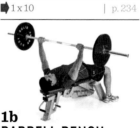

1b BARBELL BENCH PRESS ECCENTRIC
➡ 3 x 5–8 | p. 266

After the third set, add 1 drop set.

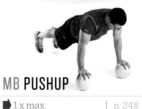

MB PUSHUP
➡ 1 x max | p. 248

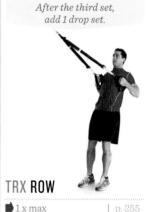

1c PULLUP
➡ 1 x max, 2 x max (Superband) | p. 235

After the third set, add 1 drop set.

TRX ROW
➡ 1 x max | p. 255

WEEK 8 MON

THE PLAYOFFS

MASTERING THE MATRIX
total-body workout

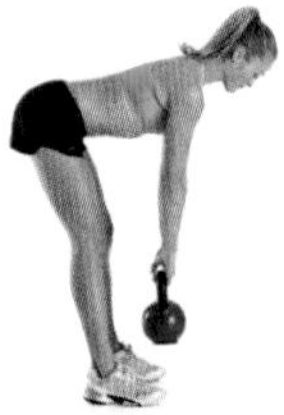

2a
KB DOUBLE-LEG ROMANIAN DEADLIFT

➡ 1 x 15, 2 x 10 | p. 252

After the third set, add 1 drop set.

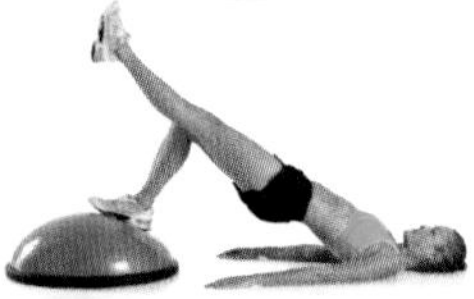

BOSU SINGLE-LEG HIP BRIDGE

➡ 1 x 15 | p. 238

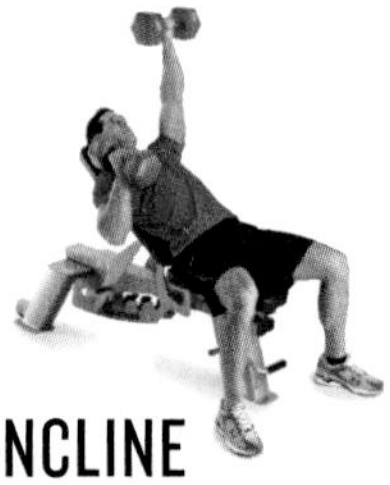

2b
DB INCLINE ALTERNATING BENCH PRESS ECCENTRIC

➡ 1 x 5–8 | p. 263

After the third set, add 1 drop set.

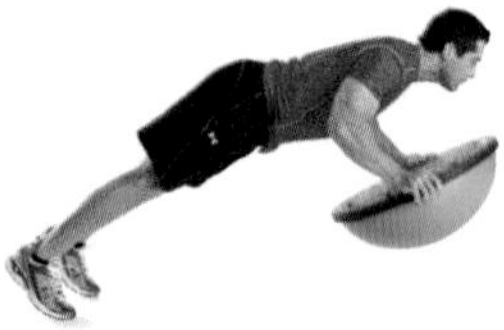

BOSU PLYO PUSHUP
DOME DOWN

➡ 1 x max | p. 240

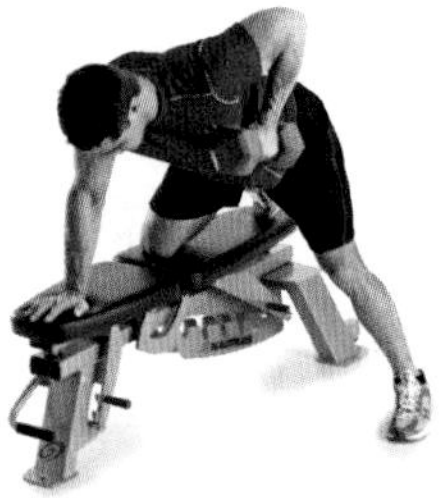

2c
DB SINGLE-ARM ROW

➡ 1 x 10, 2 x 8 / arm | p. 261

After the third set, add 1 drop set.

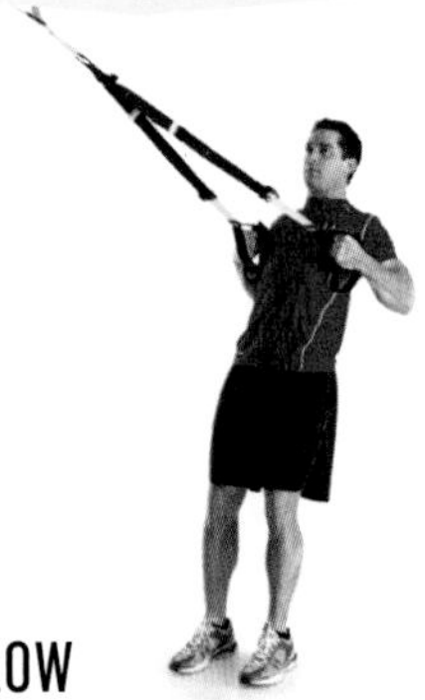

TRX ROW

➡ 1 x max | p. 255

In the Box

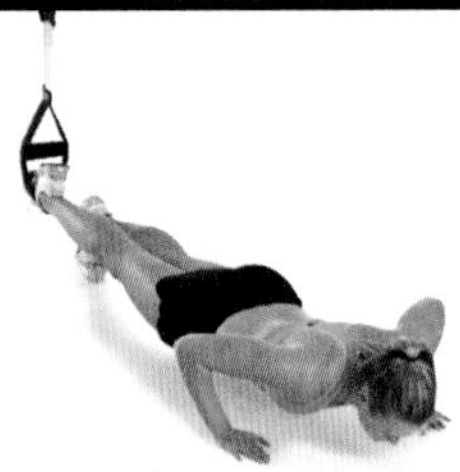

TRX BURPEE

➡ 1 x 10 / leg | p. 254

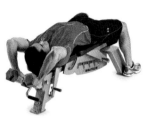

3a
DB ROLLING TRICEPS SUPERSET
➡ 2 x 10/10–15 | p. 263

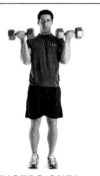

3b
DB BICEPS CURL
RUN THE RACK
➡ 2 x 5–10 / weight | p. 257

In the Box

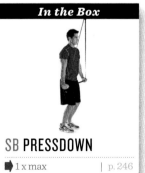

SB PRESSDOWN
➡ 1 x max | p. 246

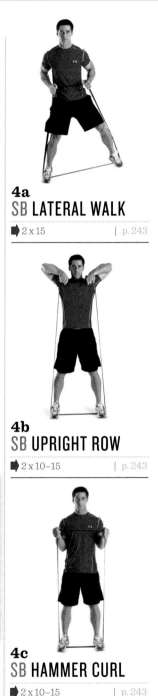

4a
SB LATERAL WALK
➡ 2 x 15 | p. 243

4b
SB UPRIGHT ROW
➡ 2 x 10–15 | p. 243

4c
SB HAMMER CURL
➡ 2 x 10–15 | p. 243

IMPACT DICTIONARY

In the Box

I love being "in the box." I use this concept in many of the fitness sessions and classes I teach. When "in the box" appears in a workout, it means that after a station is over, I want you to complete one more exercise (occasionally two exercises) with only 1 set at maximum intensity. You can take up to 60 seconds of rest after your station is completed before you begin your maximum effort "in the box." The better condition you're in, the less time you'll need before you start. This allows you to crank up the volume and diversity within your workout without adding much time. Get after it and have some fun!

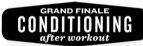

GRAND FINALE
CONDITIONING
after workout

sprint 1	**1 MINUTE ON** **1 MINUTE OFF**
sprint 2	**45 SEC ON** **45 SEC OFF**
sprint 3	**30 SEC ON** **30 SEC OFF**

1 MINUTE OFF
Repeat this circuit again.

WEEK 8 WED

THE PLAYOFFS

MASTERING THE MATRIX
upper-body emphasis

1 THE DYNAMIC WARMUP

1 JUMPING JACK	7 LUNGE & ROTATE	12 SKIPPING BACKWARD
2 GATE SWING	8 REVERSE LUNGE & REACH OVER TOP	13 FRANKENSTEIN WALK
3 POGO HOP	9 CARIOCA	14 FRANKENSTEIN SKIP
4 SEAL JACK	10 LIZARD CRAWL	15 INCHWORM
5 BODYWEIGHT SQUAT	11 SKIPPING FORWARD	16 HIP SWING
6 SIDE LUNGE		

2 JOINT INTEGRITY

Rest approximately 30 seconds between exercises.

Shoulders

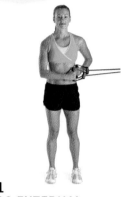

1
SC EXTERNAL ROTATION
➡ 2 x 15 / arm | p. 241

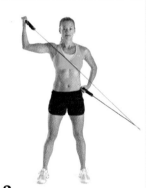

2
SC HITCHHIKER
➡ 2 x 15 / arm | p. 242

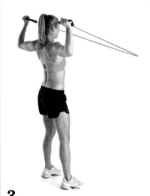

3
SC DOUBLE-ARM SCARECROW
➡ 2 x 15 | p. 242

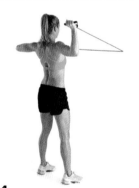

4
SC SINGLE-ARM SCARECROW
➡ 2 x max / arm | p. 241

3 CORE

Rest approximately 30 seconds between exercises.

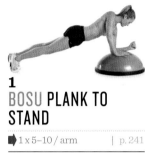

1
BOSU PLANK TO STAND

➡ 1 x 5–10 / arm | p. 241

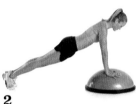

2
BOSU PUSHUP
ECCENTRIC

➡ 1 x 5–10 | p. 239

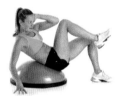

3
BOSU OPPOSITE ELBOW AND KNEE

➡ 1 x 15; 1 x 10 | p. 240

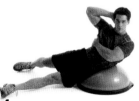

4
BOSU SIDEUP

➡ 1 x 20 | p. 237

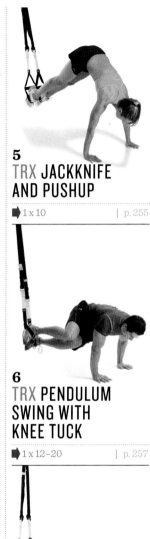

5
TRX JACKKNIFE AND PUSHUP

➡ 1 x 10 | p. 255

6
TRX PENDULUM SWING WITH KNEE TUCK

➡ 1 x 12–20 | p. 257

7
TRX PLANK

➡ 1 x 30–60 seconds | p. 254

4 STRENGTH

TRX UPPER-BODY BLAST

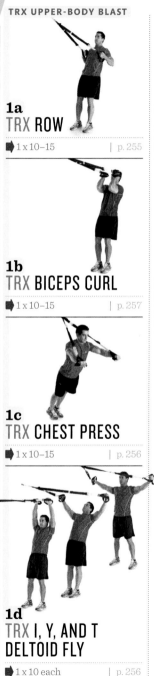

1a
TRX ROW

➡ 1 x 10–15 | p. 255

1b
TRX BICEPS CURL

➡ 1 x 10–15 | p. 257

1c
TRX CHEST PRESS

➡ 1 x 10–15 | p. 256

1d
TRX I, Y, AND T DELTOID FLY

➡ 1 x 10 each | p. 256

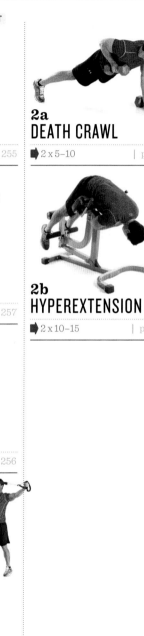

2a
DEATH CRAWL

➡ 2 x 5–10 | p. 261

2b
HYPEREXTENSION

➡ 2 x 10–15 | p. 234

WEEK 8 WED

THE PLAYOFFS

MASTERING THE MATRIX
upper-body emphasis

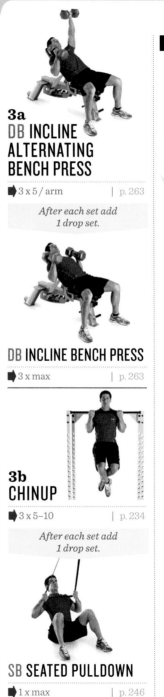

3a
DB INCLINE ALTERNATING BENCH PRESS

➡ 3 x 5 / arm | p. 263

After each set add 1 drop set.

DB INCLINE BENCH PRESS

➡ 3 x max | p. 263

3b
CHINUP

➡ 3 x 5–10 | p. 234

After each set add 1 drop set.

SB SEATED PULLDOWN

➡ 1 x max | p. 246

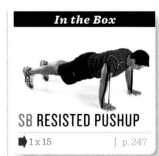

In the Box

SB RESISTED PUSHUP

➡ 1 x 15 | p. 247

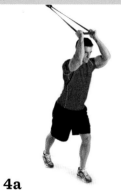

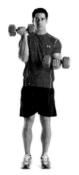

GRAND FINALE
CONDITIONING
after workout

Steady-state cardio
8-12 MINUTES
60-75% MHR

4a
SB OVERHEAD
TRICEPS EXTENSION

➡ 3 x 10–15 | p. 246

5a
BICEPS 10/10/10

➡ 1 set | p. 262

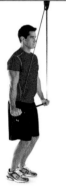

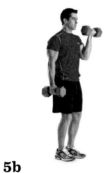

4b
SB PRESSDOWN

➡ 3 x 10–15 | p. 246

5b
DB ALTERNATING
BICEPS CURL

➡ 1 x max | p. 258

WEEK 8

THURS

THE PLAYOFFS

MASTERING THE MATRIX
lower-body emphasis

1 THE DYNAMIC WARMUP

1 JUMPING JACK	7 LUNGE & ROTATE	12 SKIPPING BACKWARD
2 GATE SWING	8 REVERSE LUNGE & REACH OVER TOP	13 FRANKENSTEIN WALK
3 POGO HOP	9 CARIOCA	14 FRANKENSTEIN SKIP
4 SEAL JACK	10 LIZARD CRAWL	15 INCHWORM
5 BODYWEIGHT SQUAT	11 SKIPPING FORWARD	16 HIP SWING
6 SIDE LUNGE		

2 JOINT INTEGRITY

Rest approximately 30 seconds between exercises.

Balance

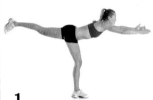

1
SINGLE-LEG BALANCE REACH-FORWARD

➡ 1 x 10 / leg | p. 230

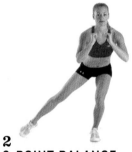

2
3-POINT BALANCE TOUCH

➡ 1 x 8–10 / leg | p. 225

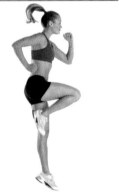

3
SINGLE-LEG BALANCE TOUCH AND HOP

➡ 1 x 10 / leg | p. 226

3 PLYOS

Complete as a circuit, repeating once. Rest approximately 30 seconds between exercises.

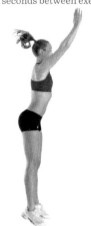

1
SQUAT JUMP WITH ROTATION

➡ 1 x 10 | p. 234

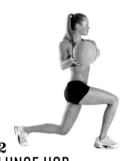

2
LUNGE HOP WITH MB ROTATION

➡ 1 x 20 | p. 250

4 CORE

3
SKATER PLYO
➡ 1 x 20 | p. 230

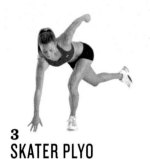

4
SINGLE-LEG
REACTIVE BOX HOP
➡ 1 x 10–15 | p. 236

1
MB SLAM
➡ 2 x 10 | p. 249

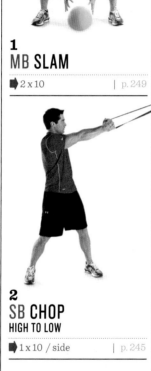

2
SB CHOP
HIGH TO LOW
➡ 1 x 10 / side | p. 245

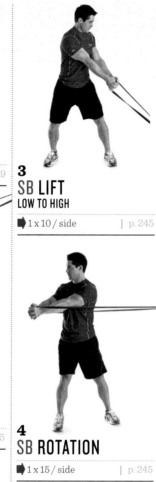

3
SB LIFT
LOW TO HIGH
➡ 1 x 10 / side | p. 245

4
SB ROTATION
➡ 1 x 15 / side | p. 245

5 STRENGTH

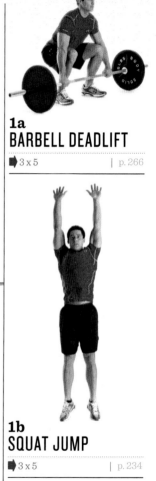

1a
BARBELL DEADLIFT
➡ 3 x 5 | p. 266

1b
SQUAT JUMP
➡ 3 x 5 | p. 234

WEEK 8 THURS

THE PLAYOFFS

MASTERING THE MATRIX
lower-body emphasis

DB COMPLEX

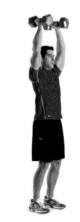

2a
DB CLEAN AND PRESS
➡ 3 x 20 | p. 259

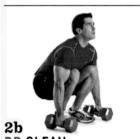

2b
DB CLEAN
➡ 3 x 10 | p. 259

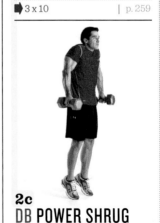

2c
DB POWER SHRUG
➡ 3 x 15 | p. 259

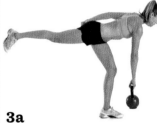

3a
KB SINGLE-LEG ROMANIAN DEADLIFT
CONTRALATERAL
➡ 2 x 10 / leg | p. 252

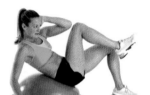

3b
BOSU OPPOSITE ELBOW AND KNEE
➡ 2 x 10 / leg | p. 240

In the Box

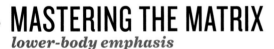

SINGLE-LEG BALANCE TOUCH
➡ 1 x 15 / leg | p. 225

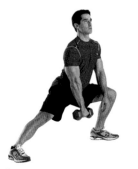

4a
DB SIDE LUNGE
➡ 2 x 15 / leg | p. 261

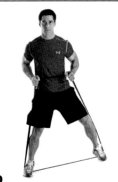

4b
SB LATERAL WALK
➡ 2 x 10–15 | p. 243

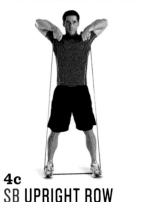

4c
SB UPRIGHT ROW
➡ 2 x 10–15 | p. 243

In the Box

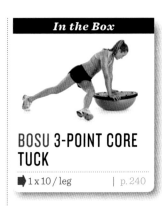

BOSU 3-POINT CORE TUCK
➡ 1 x 10 / leg | p. 240

GRAND FINALE
CONDITIONING
after workout

Sprints
80-90% of max effort
**30 SECONDS ON
30 SECONDS OFF**
6 sets

IMPACT SECRETS *from* the pros

SHAWNE MERRIMAN
LINEBACKER
SAN DIEGO CHARGERS

Todd Durkin client for 2 years

WHY HE NEEDS IMPACT TRAINING: "Todd's training is the closest thing I've seen to preparing my body for the difficulty of the NFL season. It's not about just training for strength, or just for stamina, or even becoming faster. It's about challenging your entire body so you know you got a good workout and you know you're getting better."

WHEN HE REALIZED IMPACT MADE A DIFFERENCE: "Todd pulls out these bands and the TRX, and I'm getting fatigued without even really touching the weights yet. It's crazy because I'm used to getting tired squatting 400 or 500 pounds. He'll change your mindset on what fitness is, and what fitness can do for you."

HIS TRAINING SECRET: "Bring intensity into everything you do. If you're not expecting to work out hard or aren't mentally ready to give it your all, then your mind isn't in the right place. Intensity gives you the edge in everything you do, and it's intensity that helps you achieve more."

WEEK 8

BOOT CAMP

1 TEN-MINUTE CARDIO

2 THE DYNAMIC WARMUP

1 JUMPING JACK

2 GATE SWING

3 PUSHUP

4 SEAL JACK

5 POGO HOP

6 REVERSE LUNGE
& REACH OVER TOP

7 SKIPPING

8 CARIOCA

9 FRANKENSTEIN
WALK

10 INCHWORM

CIRCUIT 1

Rest approximately 30 seconds between exercises.
Complete circuit 2 times, then run.

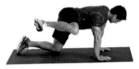

1
DIRTY DOG

➡ 1 x 15 / leg | p. 226

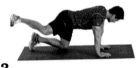

2
PUSHUP

➡ 1 x 15 | p. 229

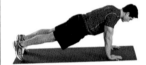

3
HORSEBACK RIDING

➡ 1 x 10 / leg | p. 227

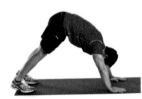

4
DIVEBOMBER
PUSHUP

➡ 1 x 10 | p. 232

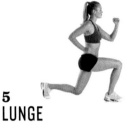

5
LUNGE

➡ 1 x 20 | p. 233

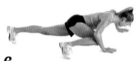

6
LIZARD CRAWL

➡ 1 x 10–20 | p. 224

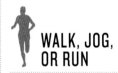

WALK, JOG,
OR RUN

➡ 3–5 minutes

CIRCUIT 2

Complete circuit 2 times, then run.

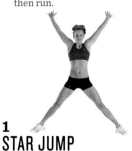

1
STAR JUMP
➡ 1 x 10 | p. 227

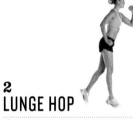

2
LUNGE HOP
➡ 1 x 20 | p. 233

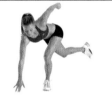

3
SKATER PLYO
➡ 1 x 20 | p. 230

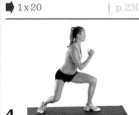

4
SURFER
➡ 1 x 10 | p. 227

RUN
➡ 3–5 minutes

CIRCUIT 3

Complete circuit 2 times, then run.

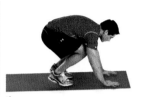

1
BURPEE
➡ 1 x 10 | p. 229

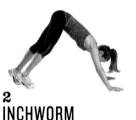

2
INCHWORM
➡ 1 x 10 | p. 224

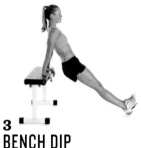

3
BENCH DIP
➡ 2 x 20 | p. 236

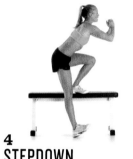

4
STEPDOWN
➡ 2 x 10–15 / leg | p. 236

RUN
➡ 3–5 minutes

CIRCUIT 4

Complete circuit 2 times.

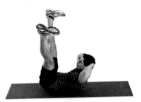

1
HELLO DOLLY
➡ 1 x 20 | p. 232

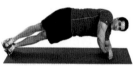

2
HIPUP
➡ 1 x 20 | p. 231

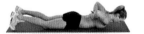

3
SWIMMER
➡ 1 x 15 | p. 230

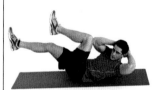

4
BICYCLE AND ROTATE
➡ 1 x max | p. 228

GRAND FINALE
CONDITIONING
after workout

300-yard shuttle run
2 MINUTES OFF
Repeat 1 time

WEEK 9 MON

THE PLAYOFFS

MASTERING THE MATRIX
total-body emphasis

1 THE DYNAMIC WARMUP

1 JUMPING JACK	7 LUNGE & ROTATE	12 SKIPPING BACKWARD
2 GATE SWING	8 REVERSE LUNGE & REACH OVER TOP	13 FRANKENSTEIN WALK
3 POGO HOP	9 CARIOCA	14 FRANKENSTEIN SKIP
4 SEAL JACK	10 LIZARD CRAWL	15 INCHWORM
5 BODYWEIGHT SQUAT	11 SKIPPING FORWARD	16 HIP SWING
6 SIDE LUNGE		

2 JOINT INTEGRITY

Rest approximately 30 seconds between exercises.

Hips

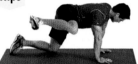

1 DIRTY DOG

➡ 2 x 15 / leg | p. 226

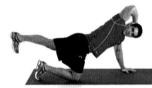

2 HORSEBACK RIDING

➡ 2 x 10 / leg | p. 227

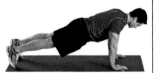

3 BIRD DOG AND ROTATE

➡ 2 x 15 / side | p. 226

4 PUSHUP

➡ 2 x 10–15 | p. 229

3 POWER

Perform circuit 2 times.

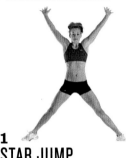

1 STAR JUMP

➡ 1 x 10 | p. 227

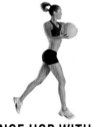

2 LUNGE HOP WITH MB ROTATION

➡ 1 x 20 | p. 250

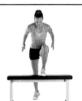

3 SKATER PLYO

➡ 1 x 20 | p. 230

4 SINGLE-LEG REACTIVE BOX HOP

➡ 1 x 10–15 / leg | p. 236

4 CORE

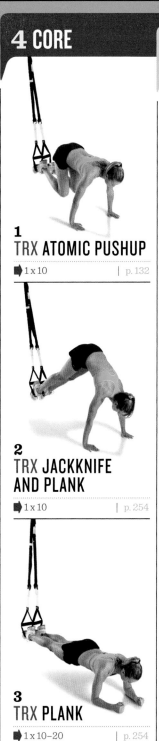

1
TRX ATOMIC PUSHUP
➡ 1 x 10 | p. 132

2
TRX JACKKNIFE AND PLANK
➡ 1 x 10 | p. 254

3
TRX PLANK
➡ 1 x 10–20 | p. 254

5 STRENGTH

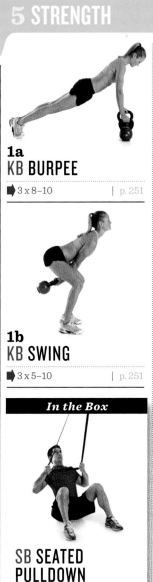

1a
KB BURPEE
➡ 3 x 8–10 | p. 251

1b
KB SWING
➡ 3 x 5–10 | p. 251

In the Box

SB SEATED PULLDOWN
➡ 1 x 15–25 | p. 246

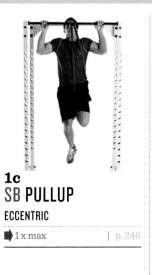

1c
SB PULLUP
ECCENTRIC
➡ 1 x max | p. 246

WEEK 9 MON

THE PLAYOFFS

MASTERING THE MATRIX
total-body emphasis

2a
TRX LUNGE
➡ 3 x 10–15 / leg | p. 253

2b
DB FLOOR PRESS
➡ 2 x 15, 1 x max | p. 264

2c
TRX ROW
➡ 3 x 10–15 | p. 255

2d
TRX BICEPS CURL
➡ 3 x 10–15 | p. 257

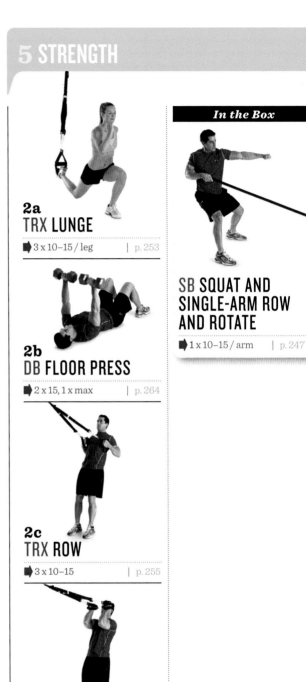

In the Box

SB SQUAT AND SINGLE-ARM ROW AND ROTATE
➡ 1 x 10–15 / arm | p. 247

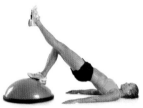

3a
BOSU SINGLE-LEG HIP BRIDGE
➡ 2 x 15 / leg | p. 238

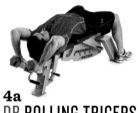

4a
DB ROLLING TRICEPS SUPERSET
➡ 2 x 8–10 | p. 263

GRAND FINALE
CONDITIONING
after workout

sprint 1   **2 MINUTES ON 1 MINUTE OFF**

sprints 2–4   **1 MINUTE ON 1 MINUTE OFF**

sprints 5–6   **30 SEC ON 30 SEC OFF**

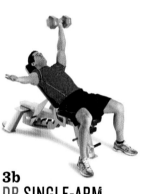

3b
DB SINGLE-ARM INCLINE BENCH PRESS
➡ 2 x 8–12 / arm | p. 263

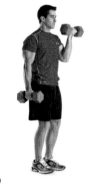

4b
DB ALTERNATING BICEPS CURL
➡ 2 x 8–10 | p. 258

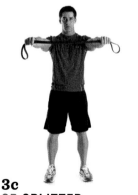

3c
SB SPLITTER
➡ 2 x 10–15 | p. 242

In the Box

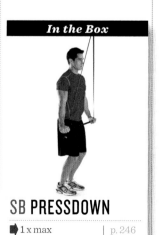

SB PRESSDOWN
➡ 1 x max | p. 246

WEEK 9 WED

THE PLAYOFFS

MASTERING THE MATRIX
upper-body emphasis

1 THE DYNAMIC WARMUP

1 JUMPING JACK	7 LUNGE & ROTATE	12 SKIPPING BACKWARD
2 GATE SWING	8 REVERSE LUNGE & REACH OVER TOP	13 FRANKENSTEIN WALK
3 POGO HOP	9 CARIOCA	14 FRANKENSTEIN SKIP
4 SEAL JACK	10 LIZARD CRAWL	
5 BODYWEIGHT SQUAT	11 SKIPPING FORWARD	15 INCHWORM
6 SIDE LUNGE		16 HIP SWING

2 JOINT INTEGRITY

Rest approximately 30 seconds between exercises.

Shoulders

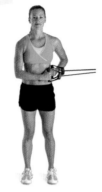

1
SC EXTERNAL ROTATION
➡ 1 x 15 / arm | p. 241

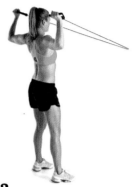

3
SC DOUBLE-ARM SCARECROW
➡ 1 x 15 | p. 242

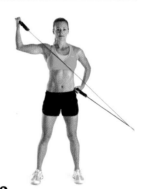

2
SC HITCHHIKER
➡ 1 x 15 / arm | p. 242

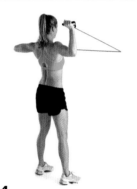

4
SC SINGLE-ARM SCARECROW
➡ 1 x max / arm | p. 241

3 CORE

Rest approximately 30 seconds between exercises.

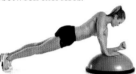

1
BOSU PLANK TO STAND

➡ 2 x 15 / arm | p. 241

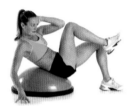

2
BOSU OPPOSITE ELBOW AND KNEE

➡ 2 x 10–15 | p. 240

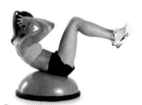

3
BOSU CRUNCH AND KICK

➡ 2 x 15 | p. 237

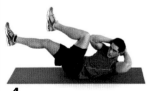

4
BICYCLE AND ROTATE

➡ 1 x max | p. 228

4 STRENGTH

TRX UPPER-BODY BLAST

Perform circuit twice.

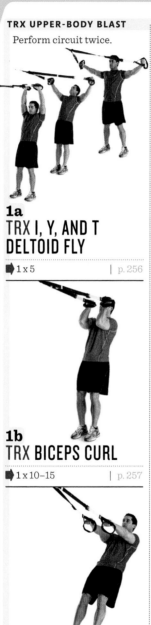

1a
TRX I, Y, AND T DELTOID FLY

➡ 1 x 5 | p. 256

1b
TRX BICEPS CURL

➡ 1 x 10–15 | p. 257

1c
TRX ROW

➡ 1 x 10–15 | p. 255

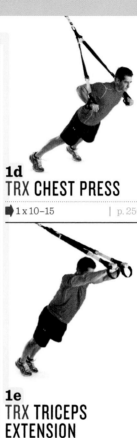

1d
TRX CHEST PRESS

➡ 1 x 10–15 | p. 256

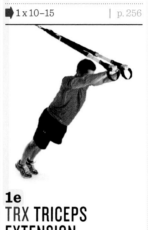

1e
TRX TRICEPS EXTENSION

➡ 1 x 10–15 | p. 255

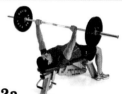

2a
BARBELL BENCH PRESS

➡ 1 x 10, 1 x 8–10, 1 x 5 | p. 266

After the third set, add a drop set.

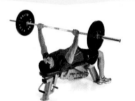

BARBELL BENCH PRESS

➡ 1 x max | p. 266

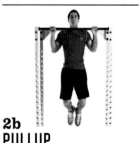

2b
PULLUP

➡ 3 x max | p. 235

After the last set, add 1 drop set.

SB SINGLE-ARM PULLDOWN

➡ 1 x max | p. 247

THE PLAYOFFS

MASTERING THE MATRIX
upper-body emphasis

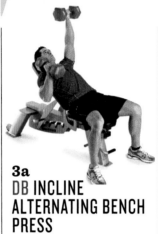

3a
DB INCLINE ALTERNATING BENCH PRESS

➡ 3 x 6–8 / arm | p. 263

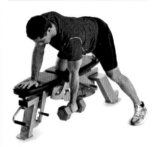

3b
DB SINGLE-ARM ROW

➡ 3 x 6–10 / arm | p. 261

In the Box

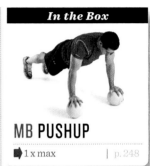

MB PUSHUP

➡ 1 x max | p. 248

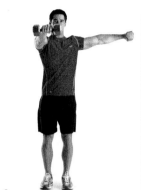

4a
DB ALTERNATING SHOULDER RAISE

➡ 2 x 8 / side | p. 258

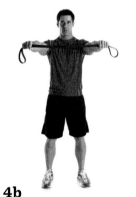

4b
SB SPLITTER

➡ 2 x 10–15 | p. 242

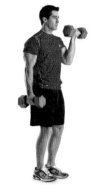

5
DB ALTERNATING BICEPS CURL
RUN THE RACK

➡ 1 x 5–10 / weight | p. 258

In the Box

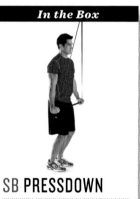

SB PRESSDOWN

➡ 1 x max | p. 246

U CALL IT!

6

➡ 5 minutes | p. 132

Steady-state cardio
8-12 MINUTES
60–75% MHR

IMPACT DICTIONARY

U Call It

"U call it" means "athlete's choice." When you see "U call it" on the workout, set your stopwatch for 5 minutes and do any exercise that is not part of the workout for that day. Complete 2 to 4 sets, depending on the exercise, and you get to determine the numbers of sets and reps. This allows you some freedom to work on areas that may need additional effort or just do exercises that you really enjoy. Have fun!

WEEK 9 THURS

THE PLAYOFFS

MASTERING THE MATRIX
lower-body emphasis

1 THE DYNAMIC WARMUP

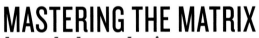

1 JUMPING JACK	7 LUNGE & ROTATE	12 SKIPPING BACKWARD
2 GATE SWING	8 REVERSE LUNGE & REACH OVER TOP	13 FRANKENSTEIN WALK
3 POGO HOP	9 CARIOCA	14 FRANKENSTEIN SKIP
4 SEAL JACK	10 LIZARD CRAWL	15 INCHWORM
5 BODYWEIGHT SQUAT	11 SKIPPING FORWARD	16 HIP SWING
6 SIDE LUNGE		

2 PLYOMETRICS

Complete circuit 2 times.

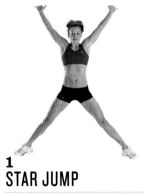

1
STAR JUMP
➡ 1 x 10 | p. 227

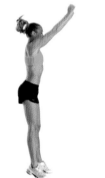

2
SQUAT JUMP WITH ROTATION
➡ 1 x 10 | p. 234

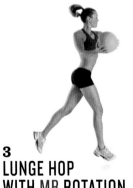

3
LUNGE HOP WITH MB ROTATION
➡ 1 x 20 | p. 250

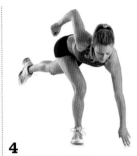

4
SKATER PLYO
➡ 1 x 20 | p. 230

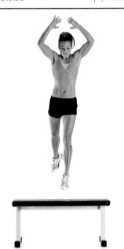

5
SINGLE-LEG REACTIVE BOX HOP
➡ 1 x 10 / leg | p. 236

3 CORE

Complete circuit 2 times.

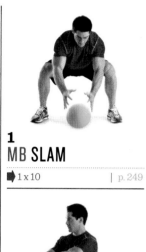

1
MB SLAM

➡ 1 x 10 | p. 249

3
SB SPLIT-SQUAT ANTIROTATION

➡ 1 x 10–15 / side | p. 244

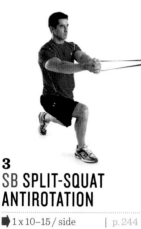

2
SB ROTATION

➡ 1 x 10–15 / side | p. 245

4 STRENGTH

DB COMPLEX

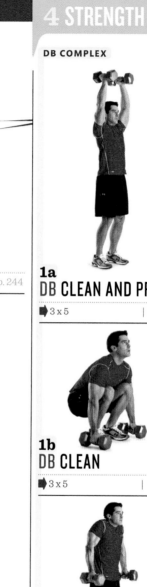

1a
DB CLEAN AND PRESS

➡ 3 x 5 | p. 259

1b
DB CLEAN

➡ 3 x 5 | p. 259

1c
DB POWER SHRUG

➡ 3 x 10–15 | p. 259

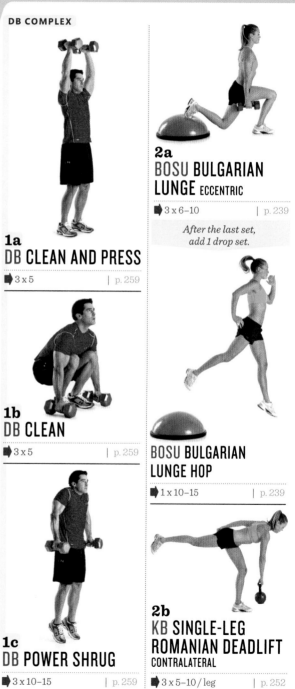

2a
BOSU BULGARIAN LUNGE ECCENTRIC

➡ 3 x 6–10 | p. 239

*After the last set,
add 1 drop set.*

BOSU BULGARIAN LUNGE HOP

➡ 1 x 10–15 | p. 239

2b
KB SINGLE-LEG ROMANIAN DEADLIFT
CONTRALATERAL

➡ 3 x 5–10 / leg | p. 252

THE PLAYOFFS

MASTERING THE MATRIX
lower-body emphasis

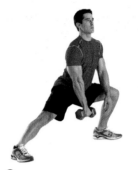

3a
DB SIDE LUNGE

➡ 2 x 10 / side | p. 261

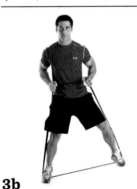

3b
SB LATERAL WALK

➡ 2 x 15 | p. 243

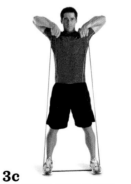

3c SB UPRIGHT ROW

➡ 2 x 10–15 | p. 243

BALANCE CIRCUIT

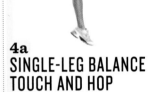

4a
SINGLE-LEG BALANCE TOUCH AND HOP

➡ 1 x 10–15 / leg | p. 226

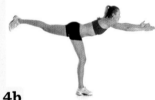

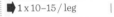

4b
SINGLE-LEG BALANCE REACH-FORWARD

➡ 1 x 10 / leg | p. 230

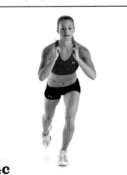

4c
3-POINT BALANCE TOUCH

➡ 1 x 10 / leg | p. 225

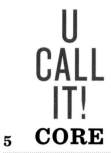

U CALL IT!

5 CORE

⏩ 5 minutes

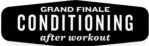

GRAND FINALE
CONDITIONING
after workout

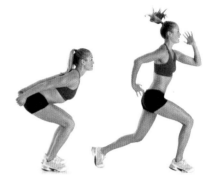

Plyo buildup

Start with 6 reps and increase until failure.

IMPACT DICTIONARY **Plyo Buildup**

Whew-eyyy! Are you ready to see how far you've come? This fitness challenge combines a squat jump and a lunge hop (see pages 233 and 234). You will complete 6 squat jumps and immediately move into 6 lunge hops. Then, without rest, you'll complete 7 squat jumps, followed by another 7 lunge hops. Keep increasing the reps until you can't go anymore (or can no longer feel your legs). Want a goal? Ten is a great number, but 15 is MVP-worthy. No one said it was easy being great!

"Remember, happiness doesn't depend on who you are or what you have. It depends solely on what you think."

— DALE CARNEGIE

WEEK 9 BOOT CAMP

1 TEN-MINUTE CARDIO

2 THE DYNAMIC WARMUP

1 JUMPING JACK	5 POGO HOP	8 CARIOCA
2 GATE SWING	6 REVERSE LUNGE & REACH OVER TOP	9 FRANKENSTEIN WALK
3 PUSHUP	7 SKIPPING	10 INCHWORM
4 SEAL JACK		

CIRCUIT 1

Rest approximately 30 seconds between exercises.

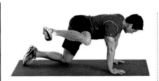

1 DIRTY DOG
➡ 1 x 15 / leg | p. 226

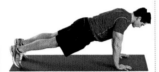

2 PUSHUP
➡ 1 x 15 | p. 229

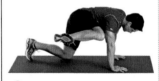

3 HORSEBACK RIDING
➡ 1 x 10 / leg | p. 227

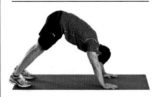

4 DIVEBOMBER PUSHUP
➡ 1 x 10 | p. 232

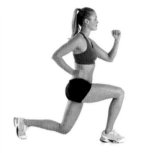

5 LUNGE
➡ 2 x 20 | p. 233

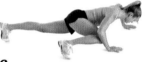

6 LIZARD CRAWL
➡ 2 x 10–20 | p. 224

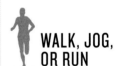

WALK, JOG, OR RUN
➡ 3–5 minutes

CIRCUIT 2

Complete circuit 2 times, then run.

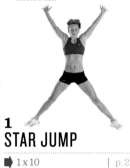

1
STAR JUMP
➡ 1 x 10 | p. 227

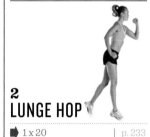

2
LUNGE HOP
➡ 1 x 20 | p. 233

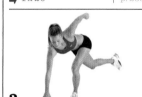

3
SKATER PLYO
➡ 1 x 20 | p. 230

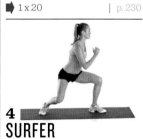

4
SURFER
➡ 1 x 10 | p. 227

RUN
➡ 3–5 minutes

CIRCUIT 3

Complete circuit 2 times, then run.

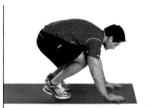

1
BURPEE
➡ 1 x 10 | p. 229

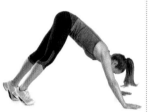

2
INCHWORM
➡ 1 x 10 | p. 224

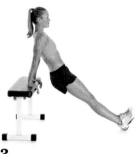

3
BENCH DIP
➡ 1 x 20 | p. 236

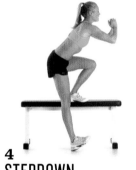

4
STEPDOWN
➡ 1 x 10–15 / leg | p. 236

RUN
➡ 3–5 minutes

GRAND FINALE
CONDITIONING
after workout

300-yard shuttle run
2 MINUTES OFF
Repeat.

CIRCUIT 4

Complete circuit 2 times.

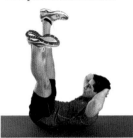

1
HELLO DOLLY
➡ 1 x 20 | p. 232

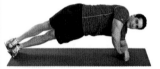

2
HIPUP
➡ 1 x 20 | p. 231

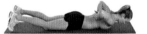

3
SWIMMER
➡ 1 x 15 | p. 230

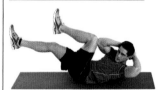

4
BICYCLE AND ROTATE
➡ 1 x max | p. 228

WEEK 10 MON

THE PLAYOFFS

IMPACT!
total-body workout

1 THE DYNAMIC WARMUP

I JUMPING JACK	7 LUNGE & ROTATE	12 SKIPPING BACKWARD
2 GATE SWING	8 REVERSE LUNGE & REACH OVER TOP	13 FRANKENSTEIN WALK
3 POGO HOP	9 CARIOCA	14 FRANKENSTEIN SKIP
4 SEAL JACK	10 LIZARD CRAWL	15 INCHWORM
5 BODYWEIGHT SQUAT	11 SKIPPING FORWARD	16 HIP SWING
6 SIDE LUNGE		

2 JOINT INTEGRITY

Rest approximately 30 seconds between exercises.

Hips + Shoulders

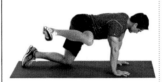

1 DIRTY DOG
➡ 2 x 15 / leg | p. 226

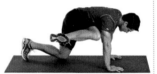

2 HORSEBACK RIDING
➡ 1 x 10 / leg | p. 227

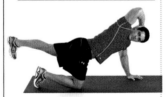

3 BIRD DOG AND ROTATE
➡ 1 x 15 / side | p. 226

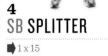

4 SB SPLITTER
➡ 1 x 15 | p. 242

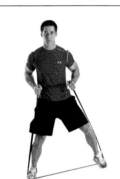

5 SB LATERAL WALK
➡ 1 x 15 | p. 243

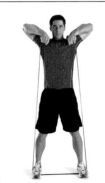

6 SB UPRIGHT ROW
➡ 1 x 15 | p. 243

Complete circuit 1 time.

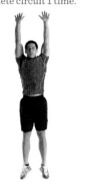

1
SQUAT JUMP
➡ 1 x 5–10 | p. 234

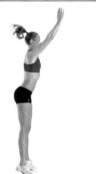

2
SQUAT JUMP WITH ROTATION
➡ 1 x 8–10 | p. 234

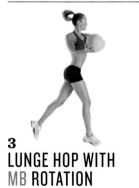

3
LUNGE HOP WITH MB ROTATION
➡ 1 x 12–20 | p. 250

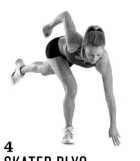

4
SKATER PLYO
➡ 1 x 12–20 | p. 230

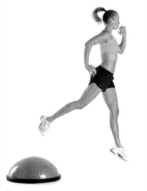

5
BOSU BULGARIAN LUNGE HOP
➡ 1 x 10–15 / leg | p. 239

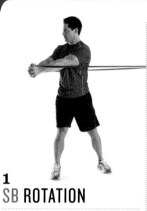

1
SB ROTATION
➡ 1 x 15 / side | p. 245

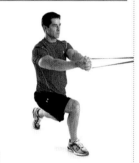

2
SB SPLIT-SQUAT ANTIROTATION
➡ 1 x 10–15 / side | p. 244

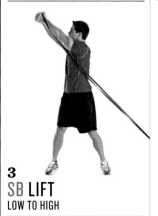

3
SB LIFT
LOW TO HIGH
➡ 1 x 10 / side | p. 245

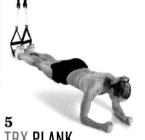

4
TRX JACKKNIFE AND PUSHUP
➡ 2 x 10–15 | p. 255

5
TRX PLANK
➡ 1 x max hold | p. 254

WEEK 10 MON

THE PLAYOFFS

→ IMPACT!
total-body workout

DB COMPLEX

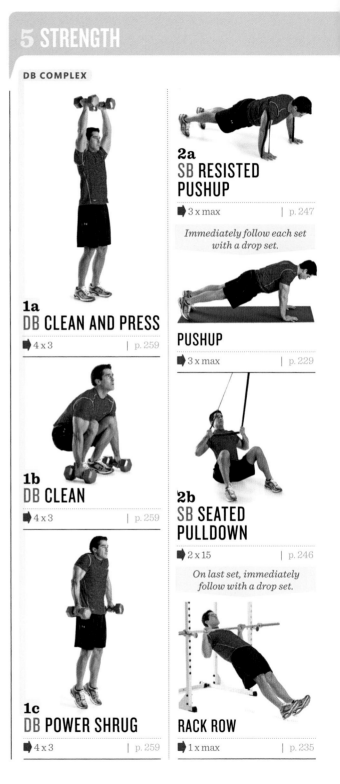

1a
DB CLEAN AND PRESS
→ 4 x 3 | p. 259

1b
DB CLEAN
→ 4 x 3 | p. 259

1c DB POWER SHRUG
→ 4 x 3 | p. 259

2a
SB RESISTED PUSHUP
→ 3 x max | p. 247

Immediately follow each set with a drop set.

PUSHUP
→ 3 x max | p. 229

2b
SB SEATED PULLDOWN
→ 2 x 15 | p. 246

On last set, immediately follow with a drop set.

RACK ROW
→ 1 x max | p. 235

In the Box

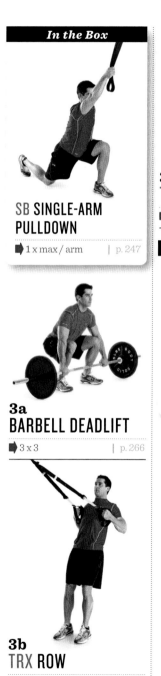

SB SINGLE-ARM PULLDOWN

➡ 1 x max / arm | p. 247

3a
BARBELL DEADLIFT

➡ 3 x 3 | p. 266

3b
TRX ROW

➡ 3 x 10–15 | p. 255

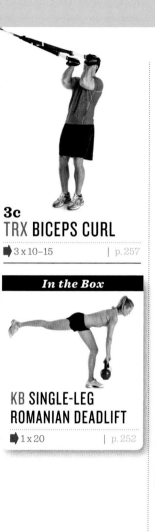

3c
TRX BICEPS CURL

➡ 3 x 10–15 | p. 257

In the Box

KB SINGLE-LEG ROMANIAN DEADLIFT

➡ 1 x 20 | p. 252

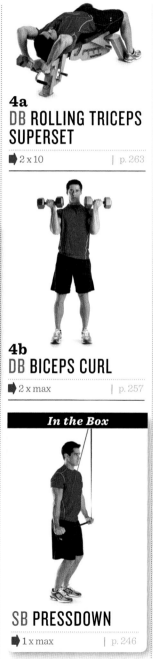

4a
DB ROLLING TRICEPS SUPERSET

➡ 2 x 10 | p. 263

4b
DB BICEPS CURL

➡ 2 x max | p. 257

In the Box

SB PRESSDOWN

➡ 1 x max | p. 246

GRAND FINALE
CONDITIONING
after workout

sprints 1-6 **1 MINUTE ON**
1 MINUTE OFF

Easy walk/jog/bike/
or your choice of cardio
3 MINUTES

sprints 2-5 **30 SEC ON**
30–60 SEC OFF

Faster speed

WEEK 10 WED

THE PLAYOFFS

IMPACT!
total-body workout

1 THE DYNAMIC WARMUP

1 JUMPING JACK	7 LUNGE & ROTATE	12 SKIPPING BACKWARD
2 GATE SWING	8 REVERSE LUNGE & REACH OVER TOP	13 FRANKENSTEIN WALK
3 POGO HOP	9 CARIOCA	14 FRANKENSTEIN SKIP
4 SEAL JACK	10 LIZARD CRAWL	
5 BODYWEIGHT SQUAT	11 SKIPPING FORWARD	15 INCHWORM
6 SIDE LUNGE		16 HIP SWING

2 JOINT INTEGRITY

Rest approximately 30 seconds between exercises.

Shoulders

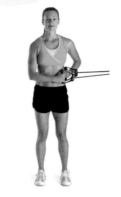

1
SC EXTERNAL ROTATION

➡ 1 x 15 / arm | p. 241

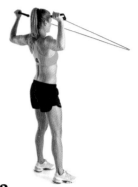

3
SC DOUBLE-ARM SCARECROW

➡ 1 x 15 | p. 242

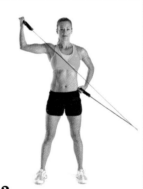

2
SC HITCHHIKER

➡ 1 x 15 / arm | p. 242

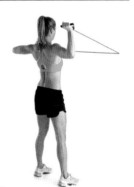

4
SC SINGLE-ARM SCARECROW

➡ 1 x max / arm | p. 241

3 CORE

Complete circuit
2 to 3 times.

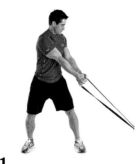

1
SB LIFT
LOW TO HIGH

➡ 2 x 10 / side | p. 245

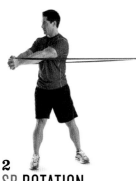

2
SB ROTATION

➡ 2 x 10–15 / side | p. 245

4 STRENGTH

DB COMPLEX

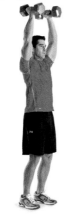

1a
DB CLEAN AND PRESS

➡ 1 x 5, 2 x 3 | p. 259

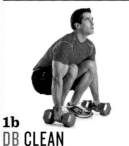

1b
DB CLEAN

➡ 1 x 5, 2 x 3 | p. 259

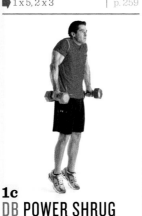

1c
DB POWER SHRUG

➡ 3 x max | p. 259

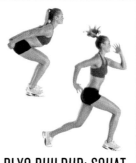

In the Box

PLYO BUILDUP: SQUAT JUMP/LUNGE HOP

➡ Start at 6 reps and build up
to 10 reps. | pp. 233, 234

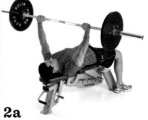

2a
BARBELL BENCH PRESS

➡ 1 x 10, 1 x 5 (eccentric),
2 x 3 (eccentric) | p. 266

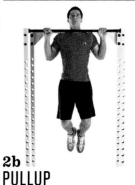

2b
PULLUP

➡ 1 x max, 3 x max (SB) | p. 235

In the Box

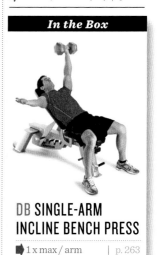

DB SINGLE-ARM INCLINE BENCH PRESS

➡ 1 x max / arm | p. 263

WEEK 10 WED

THE PLAYOFFS

IMPACT!
total-body workout

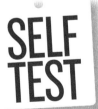

SELF TEST

After completing your Wednesday workout in week 10, take 2 days off. Then, turn to page 69 and retake the IMPACT fit test. It's time to see how far you've come.

Then, turn to page 69

4 STRENGTH

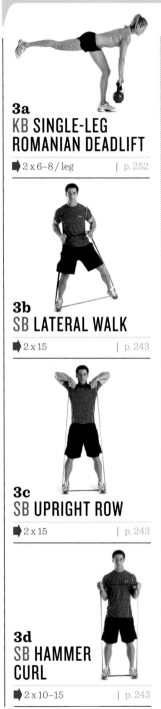

3a
KB SINGLE-LEG ROMANIAN DEADLIFT
➡ 2 x 6–8 / leg | p. 252

3b
SB LATERAL WALK
➡ 2 x 15 | p. 243

3c
SB UPRIGHT ROW
➡ 2 x 15 | p. 243

3d
SB HAMMER CURL
➡ 2 x 10–15 | p. 243

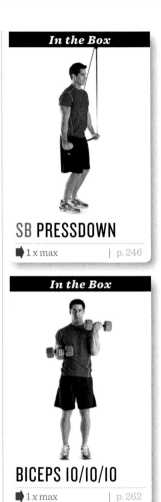

In the Box
SB PRESSDOWN
➡ 1 x max | p. 246

In the Box
BICEPS 10/10/10
➡ 1 x max | p. 262

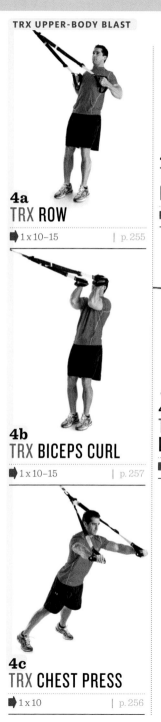

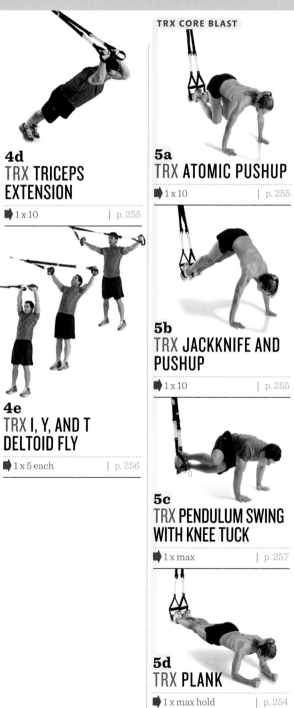

4a
TRX ROW

➡ 1 x 10–15 | p. 255

4b
TRX BICEPS CURL

➡ 1 x 10–15 | p. 257

4c
TRX CHEST PRESS

➡ 1 x 10 | p. 256

4d
TRX TRICEPS EXTENSION

➡ 1 x 10 | p. 255

4e
TRX I, Y, AND T DELTOID FLY

➡ 1 x 5 each | p. 256

5a
TRX ATOMIC PUSHUP

➡ 1 x 10 | p. 255

5b
TRX JACKKNIFE AND PUSHUP

➡ 1 x 10 | p. 255

5c
TRX PENDULUM SWING WITH KNEE TUCK

➡ 1 x max | p. 257

5d
TRX PLANK

➡ 1 x max hold | p. 254

GRAND FINALE
CONDITIONING
after workout

OFF/no running or "sprinting"

Optional light cardio
10–20 MINUTES

the EXERCISE DESCRIPTIONS

Folks, here's your exercise encyclopedia—everything you need to know to perform every move in the IMPACT program. And try this smart tip: If an exercise is new to you, and many of these probably will be, rehearse it first at one-half or one-quarter speed until you get a feel for the proper form. If it requires lifting weight, try it first with a light weight or no weight. It's very exciting to try new things, but do it with brains as well as enthusiasm. Time to get after it!

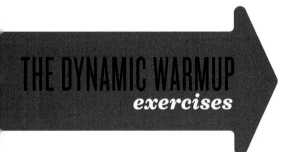

THE DYNAMIC WARMUP *exercises*

JUMPING JACK

➡ Stand with your feet together and your hands at your sides. Simultaneously extend your arms above your head and jump up just enough to spread your feet out wide. Quickly reverse the movement. Keep your ankles locked by pulling your toes up, and bounce on the balls of your feet.

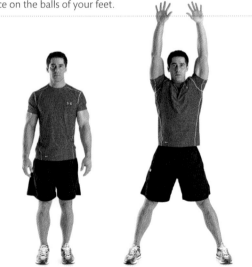

GATE SWING

➡ Stand with your feet hip-width apart and your hands at your sides. Keeping your back upright, push your hips back to lower your body into a squat. Make sure your toes point outward, and gently press your hands on your inner thighs. Hop back to the starting position.

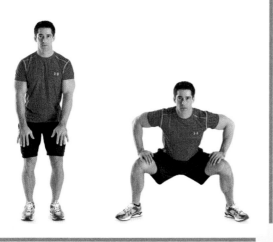

POGO HOP

➡ Stand in an athletic stance with your feet hip-width apart and your arms bent around 90 degrees. Keeping your body upright, repeatedly jump up, allowing your feet to move only a few inches from the floor. Keep your ankles locked, toes flexed up, and foot contact on the balls of your feet.

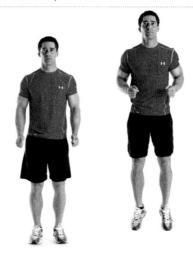

SEAL JACK

➡ Stand with your feet together and your arms extended in front of you at chest height. Simultaneously spread your arms out to the sides as you jump up just enough to spread your feet wide. Without pausing, quickly reverse the movement. Keep your ankles locked and land on the balls of your feet.

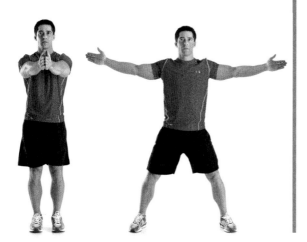

BODYWEIGHT SQUAT

➡ Stand as tall as you can with your feet spread shoulder-width apart. Lower your body as far as you can by pushing your hips back and bending your knees. Pause, then slowly push yourself back to the starting position.

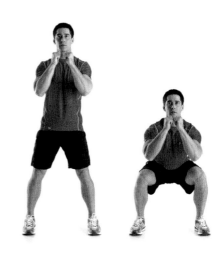

SIDE LUNGE

➡ Stand as tall as you can with your feet shoulder-width apart. Lift your left foot and take a big step to your left as you push your hips back and lower your body by dropping your hips and bending your left knee. Keep your right leg straight. Pause, then quickly push yourself back to the starting position. Repeat for desired reps before switching sides.

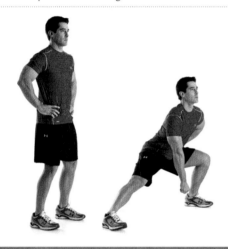

LUNGE AND ROTATE

➡ Stand tall with your feet hip-width apart, your arms extended in front of you. Step forward with your left leg and slowly lower your body until your knee is bent at least 90 degrees. Simultaneously, rotate your torso to the left. Pause, then push yourself to the starting position as quickly as you can as you rotate back to the center. Repeat with your right leg, this time twisting to the right.

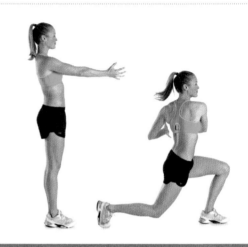

REVERSE LUNGE AND REACH OVER TOP

➡ Stand tall with your feet hip-width apart. Step backward with your left leg, and lower your body until your right knee is bent at least 90 degrees. Once in this position, reach your arms up and back toward your right shoulder. Press back up to a standing position, then step back with your right leg, this time reaching toward your left.

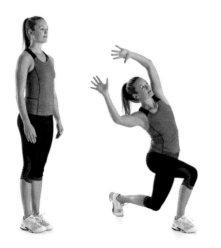

CARIOCA

➡ Assume an athletic stance with your knees slightly bent, chest up, and feet shoulder-width apart. Drive your left knee up so it crosses your right knee. Then step out with your right foot. Quickly, step your left foot behind your right, and repeat this pattern for the desired distance. It's like a moving "grapevine." Try to turn your hips with the movement but keep your chest still.

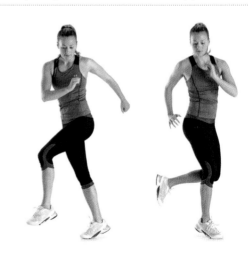

SKIPPING FORWARD

➡ Stand as tall as you can with your feet shoulder-width apart. Bring your right leg forward and up while driving off your left leg. Your left arm should move in front of your body with your elbow bent 90 degrees, while your right arm should swing back, your arm bent and hand near your rear pocket.

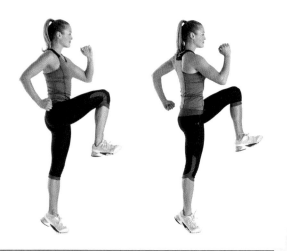

SKIPPING BACKWARD

➡ Standing tall, march backward several paces and progress into skipping backward off alternating feet. As you skip, raise your non-skipping knee toward your chest and then out away from you, opening up your hip. Then lower that foot to the ground and repeat with the other leg. Alternate legs until you cover your desired distance.

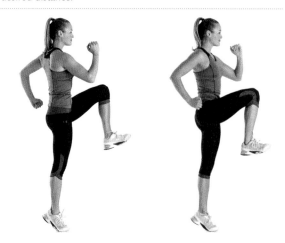

FRANKENSTEIN WALK

➡ Stand as tall as you can with your feet shoulder-width apart. Step forward with your left foot and kick your right leg in the air as high as possible while keeping the leg straight. When your leg reaches its highest point, reach forward with your left hand to meet your right foot. Repeat the same process with your left foot and right hand, and continue alternating legs.

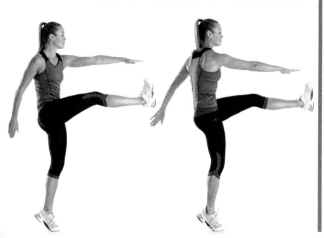

FRANKENSTEIN SKIP

➡ Complete like Frankenstein Walks, but instead of walking, add a skip between each stretch. Be sure to reach the opposite hand toward the skipping straight leg and skip off the balls of the feet.

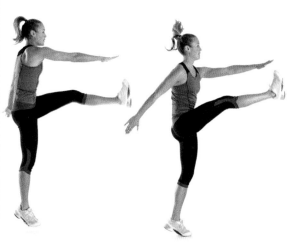

INCHWORM

➡ Stand tall with your legs straight and bend over and touch the floor. Keeping your legs straight, walk your hands forward as far as you can without letting your hips sag. Then take tiny steps to walk your feet back to your hands. That's 1 rep.

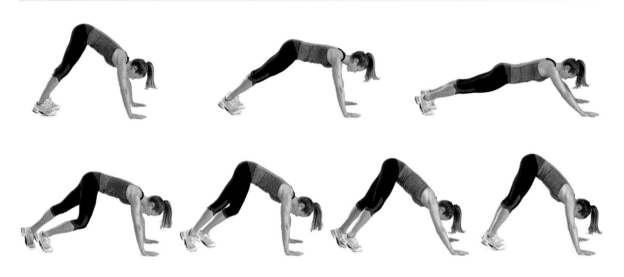

HIP SWING

➡ Stand tall and hold on to a sturdy object with your left hand. Brace your core. Keep your left knee straight, and swing your left leg forward as high as you comfortably can. Then swing it back as far as you can. That's 1 rep. Swing back and forth continuously. Complete all your reps, then switch sides and repeat.

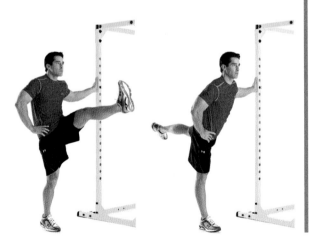

LIZARD CRAWL

➡ From pushup position on the floor, walk forward with your left arm as you lift your right foot and step forward. Now repeat with your right hand and left foot. With each step, lower your body toward the floor. Continue alternating, and keep your back straight throughout the motion. To make it more difficult, add a pushup by bringing your head close to the floor and bending your elbows after each step.

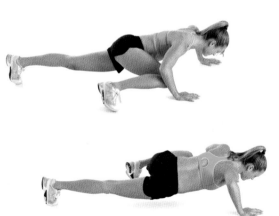

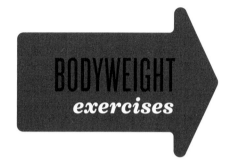

SINGLE-LEG BALANCE TOUCH

➡ Standing on your left foot with your left knee slightly bent, bend at your hips and touch the floor with your right hand while keeping your back straight. Your right leg will go back behind you as you bend forward. Return to the starting position and repeat for the desired reps. Switch legs and repeat.

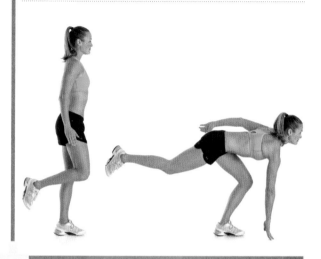

3-POINT BALANCE TOUCH

➡ Standing on your left leg with your left knee slightly bent and your chest up, bend your left knee into a quarter squat. Your right leg will have three actions without anything else moving:

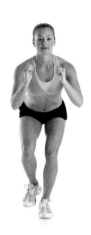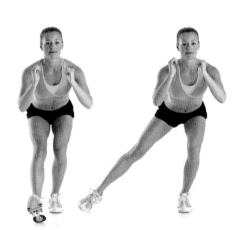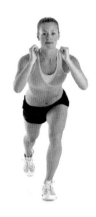

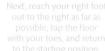

Starting position.

Reach your right foot as far forward as possible and gently tap the floor, then return to the starting position.

Next, reach your right foot out to the right as far as possible, tap the floor with your toes, and return to the starting position.

Finally, reach your right foot as far back behind you as possible, touch the floor with your toes, and return to the starting position.

That's 1 rep. The deeper you squat on your left leg, the harder it becomes. Complete all your reps, switch legs, and repeat.

SINGLE-LEG BALANCE TOUCH AND HOP

➡ Standing on your left foot with your left knee slightly bent, bend at your hips and touch the floor with your right hand while keeping your back flat. Your right leg will extend behind you as you bend forward. Then explode back up and hop off the floor. Land softly and repeat the action for the number of desired reps. Then switch legs and repeat.

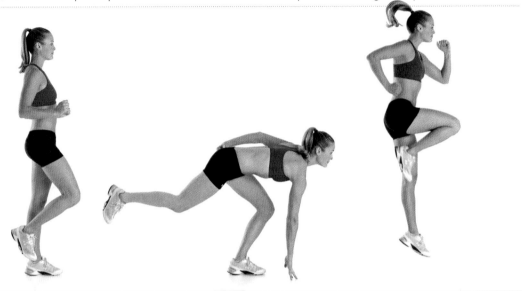

BIRD DOG AND ROTATE

➡ Get down on all fours and place your right hand behind your head. Bring your right elbow and left knee underneath your body so that they touch. Then, extend your left leg straight behind you as you rotate your torso as far as you can to the right, and return to the starting position. Complete all reps, then repeat on the other side.

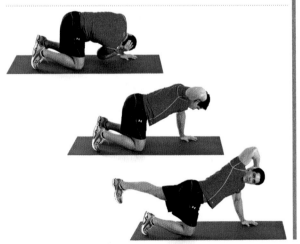

DIRTY DOG

➡ Get down on your hands and knees with your palms flat on the floor and shoulder-width apart. Relax your core so that your lower back and abdomen are in their natural positions. Without allowing your lower-back posture to change, raise your right knee and ankle straight out to the side. Keep your toes flexed toward your nose and keep your knee bent at 90 degrees. Lift your knee as high as possible. Complete all reps, switch legs, and repeat.

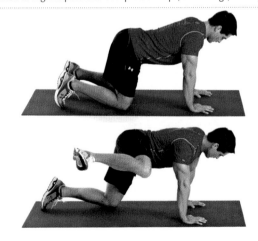

STAR JUMP

➡ With feet about shoulder-width apart, squat down so your hands are at your sides. Then, in one movement, jump up into the air and spread your arms and legs as wide as you possibly can. Return to the starting position and repeat.

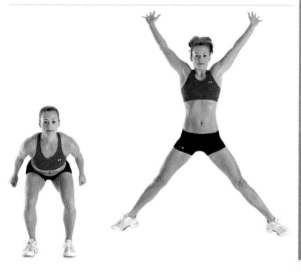

SURFER

➡ Lie flat on your stomach on the floor. In one movement, pop up to your feet and land in a surfer's position, standing up with your knees bent. Return to the starting position and repeat.

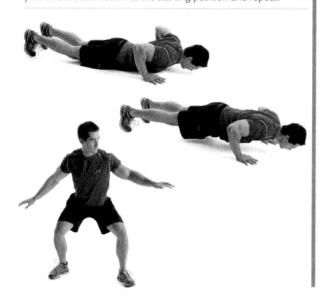

HORSEBACK RIDING

➡ Get down on your hands and knees with your palms flat on the floor and shoulder-width apart. Relax your core so that your lower back and abdomen are in their natural positions. Without allowing your lower-back posture to change, lift your hip and knee forward as if you were getting on a horse. With the same leg, then raise your hip and knee backward as if you were getting off a horse. Complete all reps with your right leg, then switch sides.

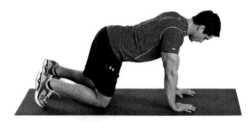

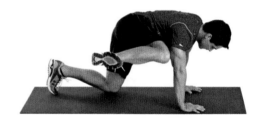

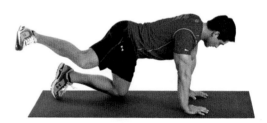

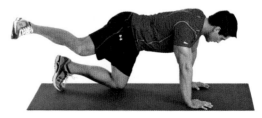

BICYCLE AND ROTATE

➡ Lie faceup with your hips and knees bent 90 degrees so that your lower legs are parallel to the floor. Place your fingers on the sides of your head. Lift your shoulders off the floor and hold them there. Twist your upper body to the left as you pull your left knee in as fast as you can until it touches your left elbow. Simultaneously straighten your right leg. Return to the starting position and repeat to the other side.

STANDING PLANK

➡ Get down on all fours and place your hands on the floor so that they're slightly wider than and in line with your shoulders. Support your weight on only your toes and hands. Your body should form a straight line from your shoulders to your ankles. Brace your core by contracting your abs as if you were about to be punched in the gut. Hold this position for the desired time.

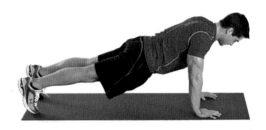

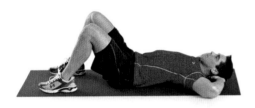

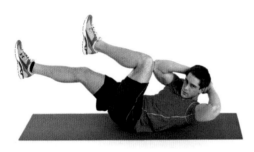

HOVER PLANK

➡ Start to get into a pushup position on the floor, but bend your elbows and rest your weight on your forearms instead of on your hands. Your body should form a straight line from your shoulders to your ankles. Brace your core by contracting your abs as if you were about to be punched in the gut. Hold this position for the desired time.

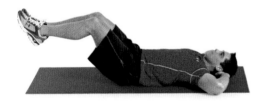

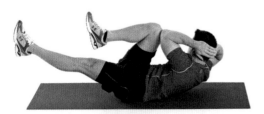

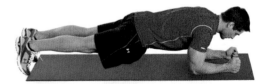

PUSHUP

➡ Get down on all fours and place your hands slightly wider than and in line with your shoulders. Support your weight on only your hands and toes. Lower your body until your chest nearly touches the floor. Pause, then quickly push yourself back to the starting position.

PLYO PUSHUP

➡ Get down into pushup position with your hands on the floor so that they're slightly wider than and in line with your shoulders. Lower your body until your chest nearly touches the floor. Pause, then push yourself up so forcefully that your hands leave the floor. Land back in the starting position and repeat.

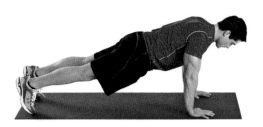

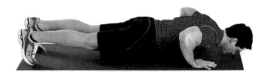

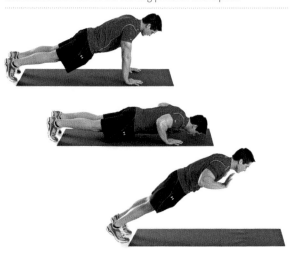

BURPEE

➡ Stand with your feet shoulder-width apart and your arms at your sides. Push your hips back, bend your knees, and lower your body into as deep of a squat as you can. Now kick your legs backward, so that you're in a pushup position. Perform a pushup, then quickly bring your legs back to the squat position. Stand up quickly and jump. That's 1 rep.

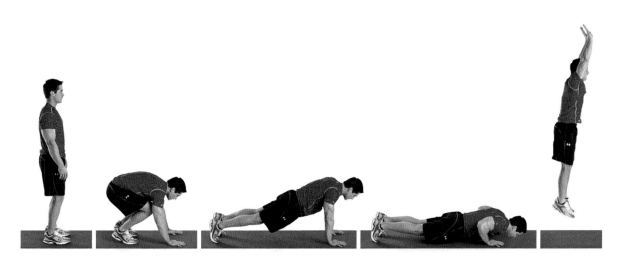

SWIMMER

➡ Lie on your stomach with your arms in front of you and over your head, palms down. Move your arms out to your sides and all the way to your hips. Glide the backs of your hands up your back as far as possible, pause, and return to the starting position.

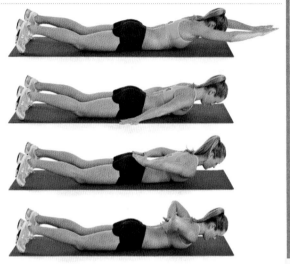

SKATER PLYO

➡ Stand on your right foot with your right knee slightly bent, and place your left foot just behind your right ankle. Bend your right knee and lower your body into a partial squat. Then bound to the left by jumping off your right foot. Land on your left foot and bring your right foot behind your left as you reach toward the floor with your right hand. Repeat the move back toward the right, landing on your right foot and left hand.

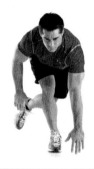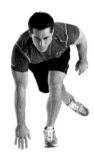

RUNNING MAN SITUP

➡ Lie on your back with your legs straight and arms at your sides, keeping your elbows bent 90 degrees. As you sit up, bring your right knee toward your chest right while you swing your right arm back and left arm forward. It should look like you're running on the floor. Lower your body to the starting position, and repeat on the other side.

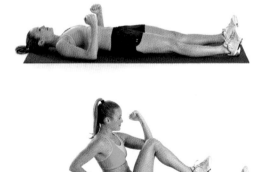

SINGLE-LEG BALANCE REACH-FORWARD

➡ Standing on your left foot with your left knee slightly bent, bend at your hips and reach forward as far as you can with both hands as your chest moves toward the floor and your right leg extends behind you. Keep your back flat throughout the range of motion. Pause and return to the starting position, and finish all the prescribed reps on that leg. Switch legs and repeat.

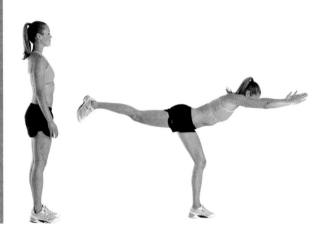

GORILLA PULLUP

➡ Grab a chinup bar with your palms facing each other and your hands about 1 to 2 inches apart. Hang at arm's length and cross your ankles behind you. Pull your left shoulder up to the bar, pause, and then lower back to the starting position. Then, repeat by pulling your right shoulder to the bar. That's 1 rep.

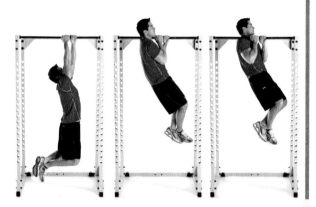

HIP BRIDGE

➡ Lie face-up with your knees bent and your feet flat on the floor. Lift your hips off the floor so your body forms a straight line from your shoulders to your knees. Drive your heels into the ground. Hold for 1 second, then return to the starting position. Repeat for the desired reps.

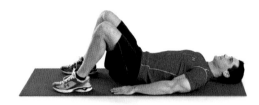

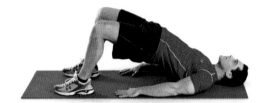

SINGLE-LEG ROTATIONAL TOUCH

➡ Stand on your right foot. Hinging from your hips and keeping your back straight, lower your upper body toward the ground. As you do so, reach your left hand toward your right foot as your left leg extends behind you. Return to the starting position and repeat for the desired reps. (To make it more challenging, start with your arms above your head.)

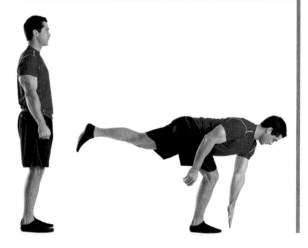

HIPUP

➡ Lie on your left side with your knees straight. Prop your upper body up on your left elbow and forearm. Raise your hips so that your torso is higher than parallel to the floor. Pause, and then lower yourself back to the starting position.

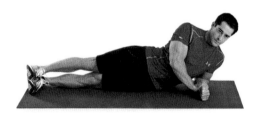

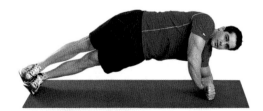

DIVEBOMBER PUSHUP

➧ Begin in standard pushup position, but move your feet forward and raise your hips so your body forms an upside-down V. Keeping your hips up, lower your body until your chin nearly touches the floor. Lower your hips until they almost touch the floor, as you simultaneously raise your head and shoulders toward the ceiling. Reverse the movement back to the starting position.

HELLO DOLLY

➧ Lie on your back with legs straight up in the air. Place your fingertips behind your ears, and pull your elbows back so that they're in line with your body. Raise your head and shoulders and crunch toward your pelvis. As you crunch up, open your legs up nice and wide. Then return to the starting position.

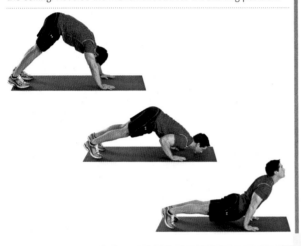

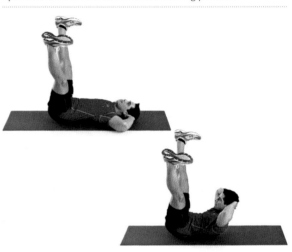

3-POINT CORE TUCK

➧ Start in pushup position, with your hands on the floor slightly wider than your shoulders. Extend your left leg as far up and to your left as possible, trying to make your toes touch your left hand. Bring your foot back to the starting position, then extend your leg under your torso toward your right hand. Return to the starting position. That's 1 rep. Do all your reps with your left leg, then switch legs.

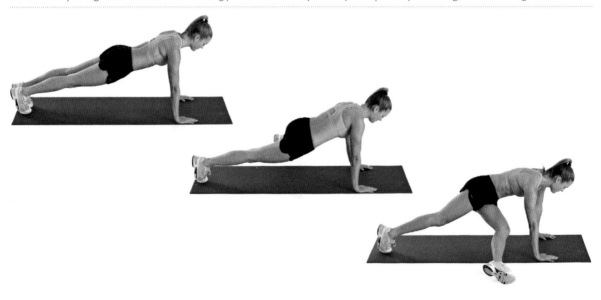

LUNGE HOP

➥ Stand in a staggered stance, your right foot in front of your left, with your arms next to your sides. Slowly lower your body as far as you can. Pause, then push back up and explosively jump with enough force to propel both feet off the ground. Once you land, immediately drop back down and repeat. Do all reps, then switch legs.

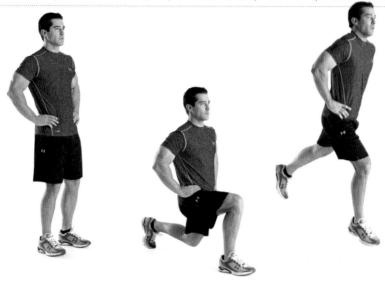

LUNGE

➥ Begin by standing normally, then step forward with your right leg and slowly lower your left leg until the knee gets close to the ground. Your right knee should bend to 90 degrees. Push yourself back up to the starting position and switch sides.

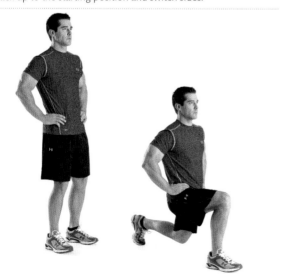

SUPERMAN

➥ Lie facedown on the floor with your legs straight and your arms next to your sides, palms down. Contract your glutes and the muscles of your lower back, and raise your head, chest, arms, and legs off the floor. At this point, your hips should be the only parts of your body touching the floor. Return to the starting position.

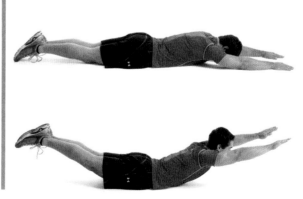

SQUAT JUMP WITH ROTATION

➡ Stand in an athletic stance with your arms at your sides. Dip your knees and squat down in preparation to leap. Explosively jump as high as you can and twist your body to the left. When you land, immediately squat down and jump again, this time rotating to the right.

HYPEREXTENSION

➡ Bend over a back extension machine with your hips fully supported and your arms crossed in front of your chest. Without rounding your back or moving your neck, raise your upper body until your chest rises just above the machine. Make sure you don't overextend your body and stress your lower back. Pause a moment, then return to the starting position. For added difficulty, hold a weight plate in front of your chest to increase resistance.

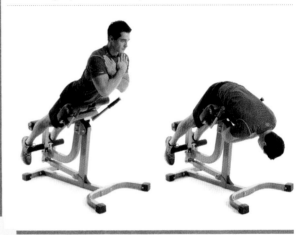

SQUAT JUMP

➡ Stand as tall as you can. Then dip your knees and squat down, swinging your arms back, in preparation to leap. Explosively jump as high as you can. When you land, immediately squat down and jump again.

CHINUP

➡ Grab a chinup bar with a shoulder-width underhand grip. Hang at arm's length, and then pull your chest to the bar. Once the top of your chest touches the bar, pause, then slowly lower your body back to the starting position.

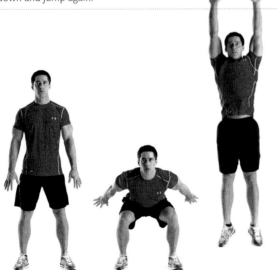

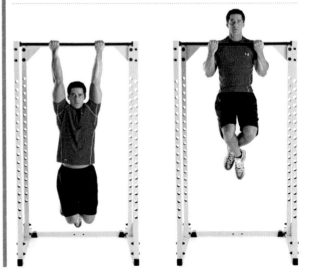

PULLUP

➡️ Grab a chinup bar using a shoulder-width overhand grip. Hang at arm's length and cross your ankles behind you. Pull your chest up to the bar. Once the top of your chest touches the bar, pause, then slowly lower your body back to a dead hang.

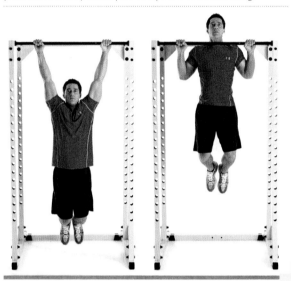

MIXED-GRIP CHINUP

➡️ Grab the chinup bar using a shoulder-width grip, with an underhand grip for one hand and an overhand grip for the other. Pull your chest to the bar. Once the top of your chest touches the bar, pause, then slowly lower your body back to the start.

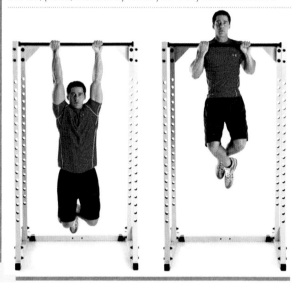

RACK ROW

➡️ Grab a secured bar (in a squat rack or Smith machine), using a shoulder-width overhand grip. Hang with your arms straight and your hands directly above your shoulders. Your body should form a straight line from ankles to head. Pull your shoulder blades back, then lift your chest to the bar. Pause, then slowly lower your body to the starting position.

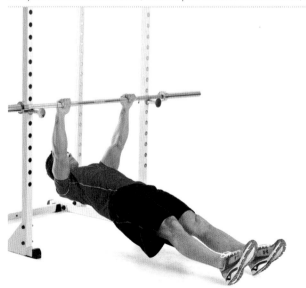

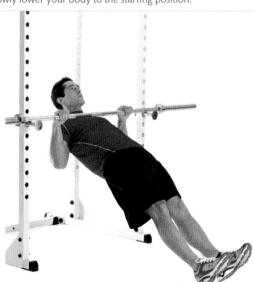

SINGLE-LEG REACTIVE BOX HOP

▶ Stand facing a bench or step that's knee height and place your left foot firmly on the step. Press your left heel into the bench and push your body up explosively so that both legs go up in the air. Land back in the starting position, with your left foot on the bench, and quickly explode up again. Complete all your reps, then switch legs and repeat.

STEPDOWN

▶ Stand on your left leg on a bench or box that's about knee height. Keeping your arms out to the side (easier) or out in front (harder), slowly lower your right leg until your right heel touches the ground. Pause, then lift yourself back up using your left leg. Repeat for the desired reps, then switch sides.

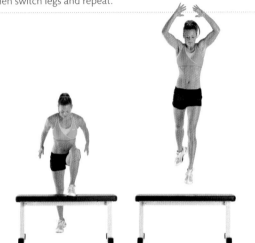

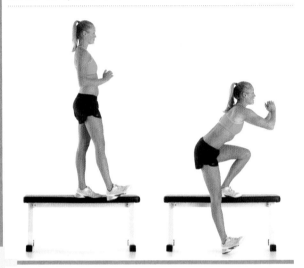

BENCH DIP

▶ Sit on a flat bench with your hands on the bench at your sides. Keep your palms on the bench at all times with your fingers facing forward and your palms down. Walk your feet out a couple of steps until your legs are extended, and lower your body just in front of the bench until your elbows are bent 90 degrees. Then press through your palms to return to the starting position.

DIP

▶ Grasp the bars of a dip station and support your weight on your hands, with your upper arms about parallel to the floor. Keeping your body upright, extend your arms until they are completely straight. Pause, then return to the starting position.

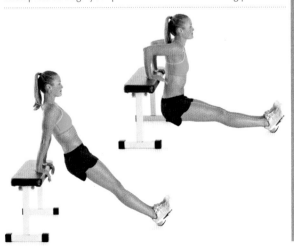

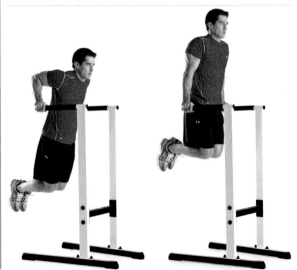

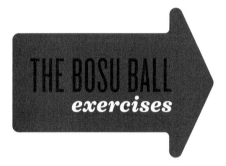

THE BOSU BALL
exercises

BOSU HIPUP

▶ Position a BOSU ball on the floor with the dome side up. Lie on your left side with your left forearm on the ball. Prop your upper body up onto your left elbow and forearm. Raise your hips until your body forms a straight line from your ankles to your shoulders. Complete a rep, then switch sides.

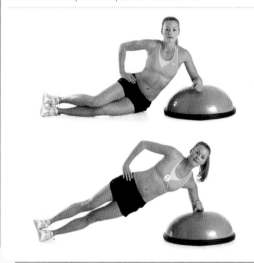

BOSU SIDEUP

▶ Lie on your left side with your hip on a BOSU dome, and with your right leg behind your left leg. Your right arm is behind your head and your left arm is across your chest. Raise your hips as high as you can, then slowly return to the starting position. Repeat for the desired reps, then switch sides.

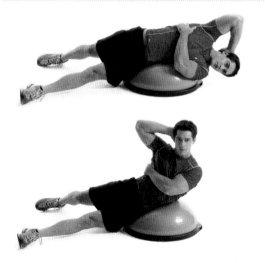

BOSU CRUNCH AND KICK

▶ Position a BOSU ball on the floor with the dome side up. Lie faceup on the BOSU with your lower back supported by the dome, your fingertips behind your ears, your elbows back, and your legs extended. In one movement, lift your torso while pulling your knees toward your chest. Lower your body to the starting position.

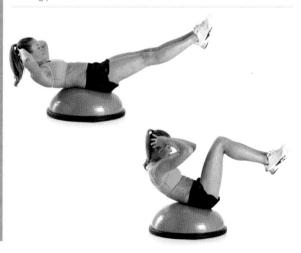

BOSU HIP BRIDGE

➡ Place a BOSU ball on the floor, dome side up. Lie faceup on the floor with your feet on top of the BOSU, your knees bent and your butt very close to the BOSU. Lift your hips up so that your body forms a straight line from your shoulders to your knees. Pause, then lower your body to the starting position.

BOSU SINGLE-LEG HIP BRIDGE

➡ Place a BOSU ball on the floor, dome side up. Lie faceup on the floor and place your left foot on top of the BOSU, with your knee bent and your right leg straight and off the floor. Push your hips up so your body forms a straight line from shoulders to knees. Pause, then lower your body back to the starting position. Do all your reps, then switch legs and repeat.

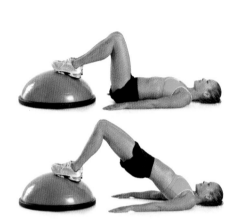

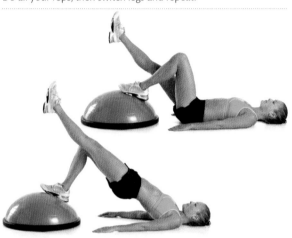

BOSU PLYO PUSHUP

➡ Place a BOSU ball on the floor, dome side up. Place your hands on top of the BOSU so that they're slightly wider than and in line with your shoulders. Lower your body until your chest touches the BOSU. Then push yourself up so forcefully that your hands leave the BOSU. Land back in the starting position.

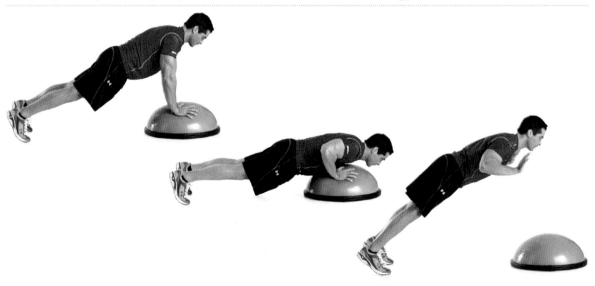

BOSU PUSHUP

➡ Place a BOSU ball on the floor with the dome side facing up. Put your hands on top of the ball and get into pushup position. Your body should form a straight line from your shoulders to your ankles. Lower your body until it's about an inch above the ball, and then quickly press back up to the starting position.

BOSU BULGARIAN LUNGE

➡ Place a BOSU ball on the floor, dome side up. Hold a pair of dumbbells at your sides and stand in a staggered stance. Place the ball of your right foot on the top of the BOSU. Lower your body as far as you can without allowing your right knee to touch the floor. Pause, then push yourself back up to the starting position as quickly as you can. Complete all the prescribed reps, then switch legs and repeat.

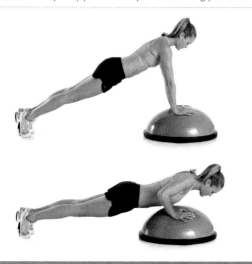

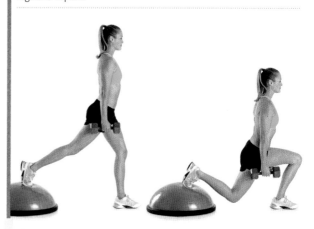

BOSU BULGARIAN LUNGE HOP

➡ Place a BOSU ball on the floor, dome side up. Stand in a staggered stance with your arms at your sides. Place the ball and toes of your right foot on top of the BOSU. Lower your body as far as you can without allowing your knee to touch the floor. Pause, then explosively push yourself up so that both feet leave the floor as you swing your arms up in the air. Land back in the starting position, regain your balance, and repeat. Complete all your reps, then switch legs and repeat.

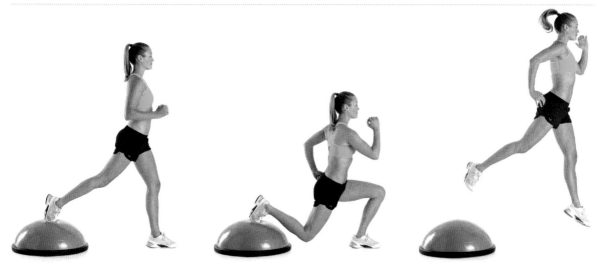

BOSU PLYO PUSHUP (DOME DOWN)

➡ Place a BOSU ball on the floor, with the dome side down. Grasp the sides of the BOSU, then lower your body until your chest nearly touches the BOSU. Pause, then explosively push your body up and pull the ball off the floor. Land, reset, and repeat for desired reps.

BOSU OPPOSITE ELBOW AND KNEE

➡ Position a BOSU ball with the dome side up. Lie with your lower back supported on top of the dome, your left hand resting behind your head, and your right leg extended. Place your right hand on the ground. Simultaneously bring your right knee and left elbow together and hold for a second. Return to the starting position, then switch sides and repeat.

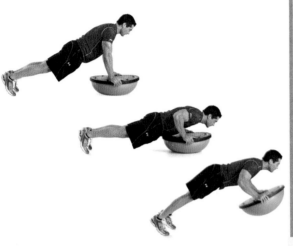

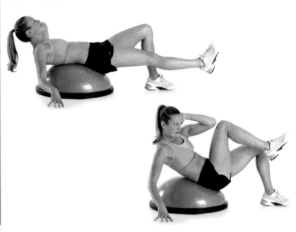

BOSU 3-POINT CORE TUCK

➡ Place a BOSU ball on the floor, dome side down. Grasp the BOSU on both sides and get in pushup position. Extend your left leg as far out to your left as possible, trying to make your toes touch your left hand. Bring your foot back to the starting position, then extend your leg under your torso toward your right hand. Return to the starting position, complete your reps with that leg, then switch legs.

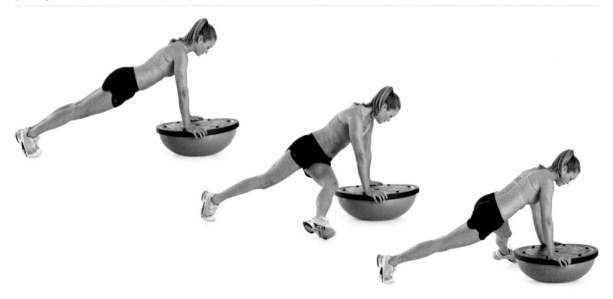

BOSU PLANK TO STAND

➡ Place a BOSU ball on the floor with the dome side up. Start in a hover plank position with your elbows and forearms resting on the BOSU. Your body should form a straight line from shoulders to ankles. Brace your core by contracting your abs as if you were about to be punched in the gut. Then extend your arms—one at a time—so that you're in pushup position on top of the BOSU. Pause, then slowly return to the starting position. That's 1 rep.

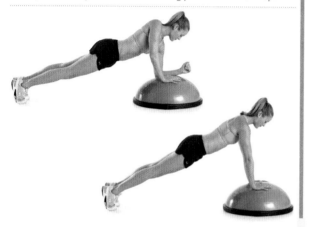

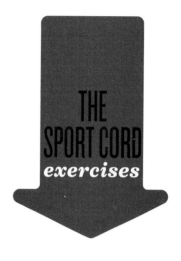

THE SPORT CORD *exercises*

SPORT CORD SINGLE-ARM SCARECROW

➡ Secure a Sport Cord to a stable object. Hold a handle in each hand while facing the anchor, and step back until you feel tension in the cords. Bend both arms 90 degrees, and raise your arms so your palms face down. Rotate your right forearm up and back as far as you can. Hold, then return to the starting position. Complete all reps on your right arm, and then repeat on your left.

SPORT CORD EXTERNAL ROTATION

➡ Secure a Sport Cord around a stable object and hold one handle in each hand. Stand with your left shoulder 2 to 3 feet away from the anchor point, bend your right elbow 90 degrees, and tuck it against your torso. Without changing the bend in your elbow, open and close your arm as far as it will go for desired reps. Switch arms and repeat.

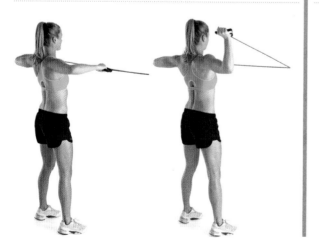

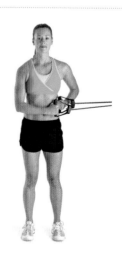

SPORT CORD HITCHHIKER

➡ Secure a Sport Cord around a stable object and hold a handle in each hand. Stand with your right shoulder about 2 to 3 feet from the anchor. Bring your left arm down and across your body so that your left thumb is reaching toward your right hip. Extend your left arm, hand, and thumb up and away above your shoulder. Repeat back and forth. Then switch arms and repeat.

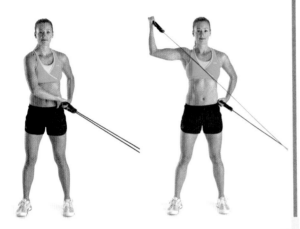

SPORT CORD DOUBLE-ARM SCARECROW

➡ Secure a Sport Cord around a stable object and hold a handle in each hand while facing the anchor. Step back so you feel tension in the cords, bend both arms 90 degrees, then raise your arms so your palms are facing down and your forearms are parallel to the floor. Without changing the position of your upper arms, rotate your forearms up and back as far as you can. Pinch your shoulder blades, hold, and return to the starting position.

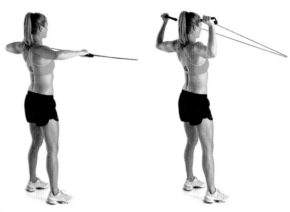

SUPERBAND SPLITTER

➡ Grab a Superband in both hands and hold the ends more than shoulder-width apart. Raise your arms so that the band is in front of your chest at arm's length. Then pull each end as far as you can, as if you're trying to snap the band in half. As you pull back, squeeze your shoulder blades together. Hold, and then return your hands slowly to the starting position.

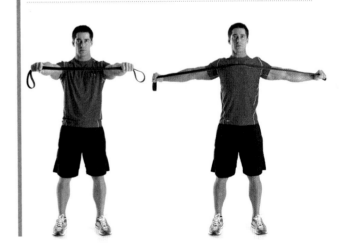

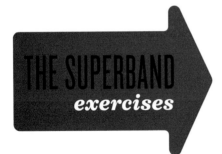

THE SUPERBAND *exercises*

SUPERBAND LATERAL WALK

➡ Grab a Superband and stand on one end with both feet about shoulder-width apart. Hold the other end of the band with both hands, your palms facing downward. Take small steps to your left for the prescribed number of reps. Then sidestep back to your right for an equal number of reps. That's 1 set.

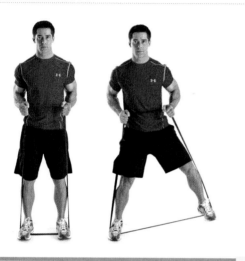

SUPERBAND UPRIGHT ROW

➡ Grab a Superband and stand on one end with your feet about shoulder-width apart. Hold the other end of the band with both hands, your palms facing your thighs. Pull the band up toward your chest and squeeze your shoulder blades together. Your elbows should point outward and move just above your shoulders. Pause, then return to the starting position.

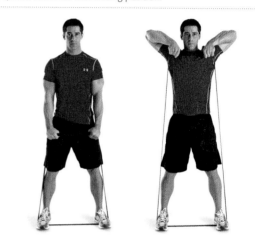

SUPERBAND HAMMER CURL

➡ Grab a Superband and stand on one end with both feet less than shoulder-width apart. Hold the other end of the band with both hands, palms facing each other. Without moving your upper arms, bend your elbows and pull the bands as close to your shoulders as you can. Pause, then slowly lower the band to the starting position. To make it easier, hold the band closer to your face. To make it harder, hold it farther from you.

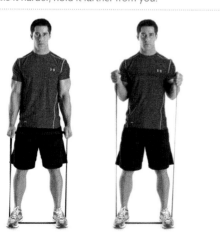

SUPERBAND FACE PULL

➡ Attach a Superband to a stable object at face height. Facing the anchor point, stand tall and keep your chest out. Grasping the Superband with both hands, arms straight, pull the band back toward your forehead, imagining that you're pinching a coin between your shoulder blades as you finish with the band in front of your face. Return to the starting position. That's 1 rep.

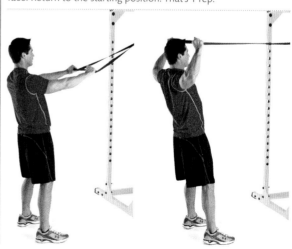

SUPERBAND ½-KNEELING LIFT (LOW TO HIGH)

➡ Attach a Superband to a stable object at ankle height. Kneel on your left knee with your left side facing the anchor. Clasp the band with both hands, turn toward the anchor, and pull the band up and across your body, and out in front of your right shoulder. Pause, then return to the starting position. Complete all reps, then switch sides and repeat.

SUPERBAND ½-KNEELING CHOP (HIGH TO LOW)

➡ Attach a Superband to a stable object above your head, such as a chinup bar. Kneel on your left knee with your left side facing the anchor. Clasp your hands around the band, and rotate so your torso faces the anchor. Pull the band down and across your body to your left hip. Pause, then return to the starting position. Do all reps, switch sides, and repeat.

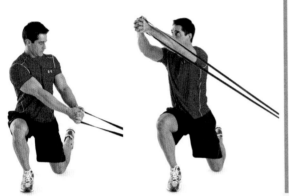

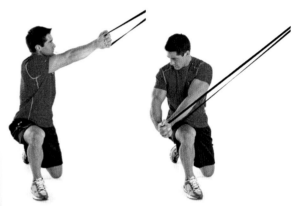

SUPERBAND STANDING ANTIROTATION

➡ Attach a Superband to a stable object at chest level. Grab the Superband with a clasped grip and stand with your left side facing the anchor point. Step away from the anchor so the cable is taut. Hold the handle against your chest. Slowly press your arms in front of you until they're straight, pause for a second, and bring them back. Do not allow any rotation. Do all your reps, then turn around and work your other side.

SUPERBAND SPLIT-SQUAT ANTIROTATION

➡ Attach a Superband to a stable object at chest height. Clasp the band with both hands and stand so that your left side faces the anchor, holding the band in front of your chest. Step away until you feel tension trying to rotate your torso toward the anchor, while you resist any movement. This is the starting position. Without rotating, press the band in front of your chest by extending your arms, pause, then return to the starting position.

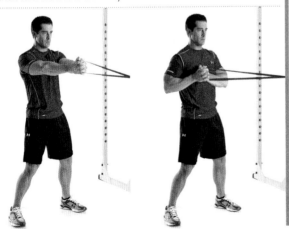

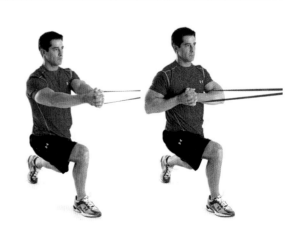

SUPERBAND LIFT (LOW TO HIGH)

➡ Attach a Superband to a stable object near your ankles. Clasp the band with both hands, and stand so that your left side faces the anchor. Keeping arms extended, rotate from approximately the knees up to your shoulder. Pause, then return to the starting position. Complete all reps to your right side, then do the same number of repetitions with your right side facing the anchor point.

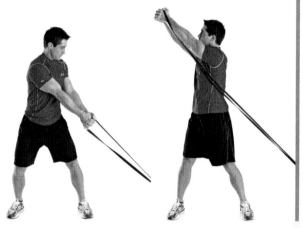

SUPERBAND CHOP (HIGH TO LOW)

➡ Attach a Superband to a stable object above your head, such as a chinup bar. Clasp both hands around the band, and step away so that your left side faces the anchor point. Your shoulders should be turned toward the band. In one movement, while keeping your arms straight, rotate your torso down and across your body so your hands end up outside your right hip. Pause, then return to the starting position. Do all reps to your right side, then repeat with your left side facing the anchor point.

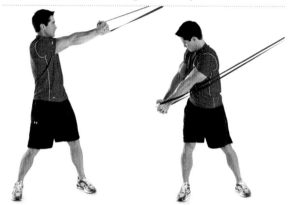

SUPERBAND ROTATION

➡ Attach a Superband to a stable object at waist height to your left. Clasp the band with both hands, and extend your arms in front of your chest, rotating your torso so that your chest faces the anchor point. In one movement, rotate your body to the right and pull the band across your body. Pause, then return to the starting position. Complete all reps to your right side, then repeat on your left side.

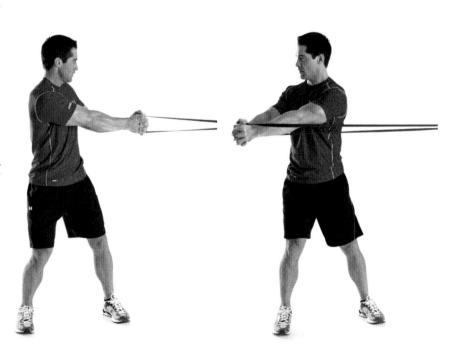

SUPERBAND PULLUP

➡ Loop a Superband around a chinup bar and pull it through so you create a knot. Grab the bar with a shoulder-width overhand grip, and place one knee in the loop of the band, and hang at arm's length. Bend your arms to pull your chest to the bar. Once the top of your chest touches the bar, pause, then lower your body to the starting position.

SUPERBAND PRESSDOWN

➡ Wrap a Superband to a secure object overhead. Grab the band with each hand, and stand facing the anchor point, just a few inches away. Bend your arms and grab the ends of the Superband with your palms facing each other. Tuck your upper arms next to your sides. Without moving your upper arms, push the band down until your elbows are locked. Slowly return to the starting position.

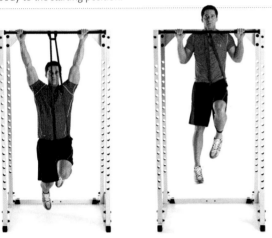

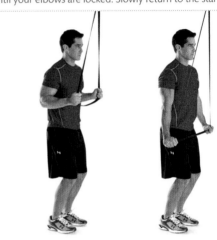

SUPERBAND SEATED PULLDOWN

➡ Attach a Superband to a stable object above your head, such as a chinup bar. Grasp the band with both hands. Position yourself 2 feet behind the anchor point and sit on the floor. Lean back slightly, then pull the band toward your chest with both hands, imagining that you're pinching a coin between your shoulder blades as you finish with the band in front of your upper chest. Return to the starting position and repeat for the desired reps.

SUPERBAND OVERHEAD TRICEPS EXTENSION

➡ Attach a Superband to a secure object overhead. Grab the band with each hand, with your back to the anchor point. Stand in a staggered stance, one foot in front of the other. Hold the band behind your head, with each elbow bent 90 degrees. Without moving your upper arms, push your forearms forward until your elbows are locked. Pause, then return to the starting position.

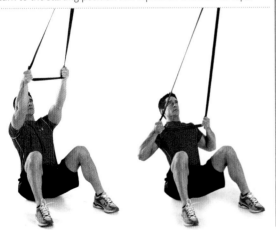

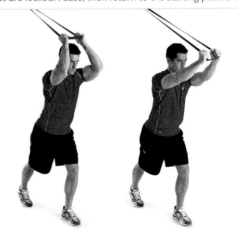

SUPERBAND SINGLE-ARM PULLDOWN

➡ Secure a Superband around a high fixed object, such as a chinup bar. Grab the end of the band with your right hand and step back until you feel tension in your back. Then kneel on your right knee, with your left knee forward and left foot flat on the floor. Pull the band to the side of your chest and squeeze your shoulder blade. Do all your reps, then switch arms and legs, and repeat the movement.

SUPERBAND RESISTED PUSHUP

➡ Grab a Superband and hold an end in each hand, with the band wrapped around your back. Still holding the band, get into pushup position. Your body should form a straight line from your ankles to your head, and the band should feel taut and pressed against your upper back, while anchored under each hand. Lower yourself until your chest is just above the floor. As you push your body up, you should feel extra resistance from the band.

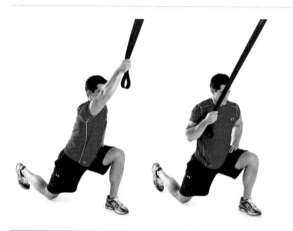

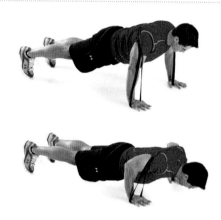

SUPERBAND SQUAT AND SINGLE-ARM ROW AND ROTATE

➡ Secure a Superband to a stable object at knee height. Grab the band with your right hand and step away from the anchor point until you feel tension. Lower your body into a squat, and extend your arm out in front of your torso. As you stand up, pull the band to the side of your chest and slightly rotate. Do all reps on one side, and then switch sides.

SUPERBAND ½-KNEELING PULLDOWN

➡ Attach a Superband to a stable object above your head, such as a chinup bar. Grasp the band with both hands. Position yourself 2 feet behind the anchor point and lower yourself to one knee. Pull the band toward your chest with both hands, imagining that you're pinching a coin between your shoulder blades as you finish with the band in front of your upper chest. Return to the starting position and repeat for the desired reps.

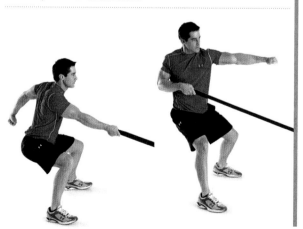

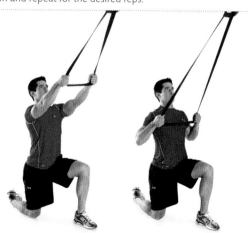

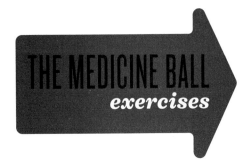

THE MEDICINE BALL *exercises*

MEDICINE BALL SINGLE-ARM PUSHUP

➡ Position a medicine ball on the floor. Place your right hand on the medicine ball and your left hand on the floor and assume a pushup position, with your body forming a straight line from your ankles to your head. Lower your body as far as you can, pause, and then press back to the starting position as quickly as possible. Roll the ball to your left hand and repeat.

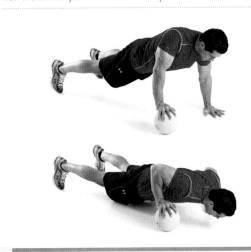

MEDICINE BALL PUSHUP

➡ Position two medicine balls on the floor, slightly wider than and in line with your shoulders. Place your hands on the medicine balls and assume a pushup position, with your body forming a straight line from your ankles to your head. Lower your body as far as you can, pause, and then press back to the starting position as quickly as possible.

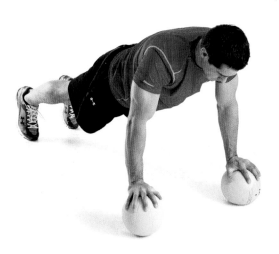

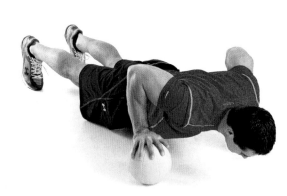

MEDICINE BALL SLAM

➡ Place a heavy medicine ball on the floor in front of you. Stand with your feet a little wider than shoulder width and your toes pointed out at a slight angle. Bend at your hips and knees and grab the ball. Without allowing your lower back to round, pull your torso back and up, thrust your hips forward, and stand up with the ball at chest level. Press the ball overhead, then slam it to the ground. Drop your hips to the starting position as you slam.

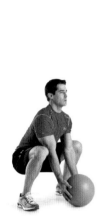
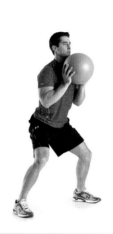
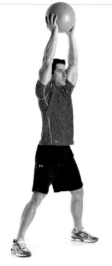
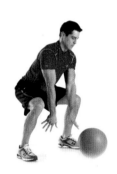

MEDICINE BALL DIAGONAL LUNGE WITH PRESS

➡ Grab a medicine ball and hold it in front of your chest with your elbows bent 90 degrees. Step forward diagonally with your left leg at a 45-degree angle as you extend your arms and press the medicine ball straight out from your chest. Walk forward to return to a base stance, then step diagonally to the right at 45 degrees and press the medicine ball forward. That's 1 rep.

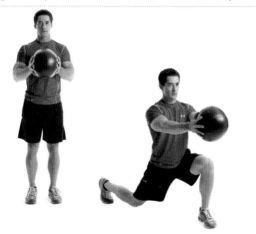

MEDICINE BALL GROUND PUSH SLAM

➡ Place a medicine ball on the floor. Squat down to pick it up, lift the ball to your chest, and jump up. On the way down from the jump, push the ball explosively down into the floor about 6 to 12 inches in front of your face. Catch the ball and repeat.

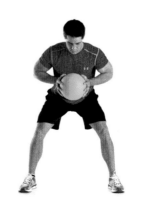
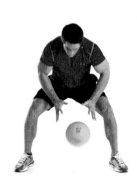

LUNGE HOP WITH MEDICINE BALL ROTATION

➡ Hold a medicine ball in front of your chest and stand with your left foot staggered in front of your right. Slowly lower your body as far as you can. Pause, then jump with enough force to propel both feet off the floor. Switch your legs as you jump, so your right leg moves forward and your left moves back. As you land, rotate your body to the right. Lower your body into a lunge and jump again, this time rotating to your left.

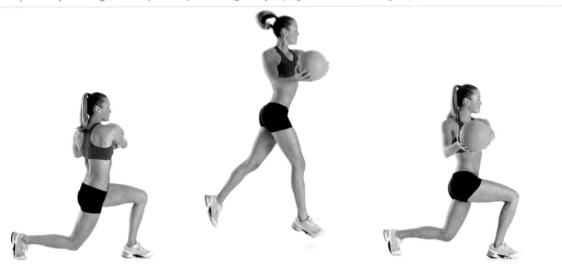

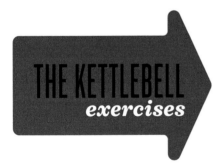

THE KETTLEBELL *exercises*

KETTLEBELL PUSHUP

➡ Place a pair of kettlebells on the floor. Get into pushup position and grab the weights so they're slightly wider than and in line with your shoulders. Your body should form a straight line from your ankles to your head. Lower your body until your upper arms are parallel to the floor, pause, and then push yourself back up.

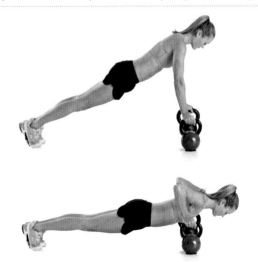

KETTLEBELL GOBLET SQUAT

➡ Hold a kettlebell close to your chest, with both hands grasping the kettlebell. Lower your body as far as you can by pushing your hips back and bending your knees. Your elbows should point down. Pause, then push back to the starting position.

KETTLEBELL SWING

➡ Grab a kettlebell with an overhand grip and hold it at arm's length. Bend at your hips and knees and lower your torso until it forms a 45-degree angle to the floor. Swing the kettlebell between your legs. Keeping your arm straight, thrust your hips forward, straighten your knees, and swing the kettlebell up to chest level as you rise to standing position. Repeat this pattern for all reps.

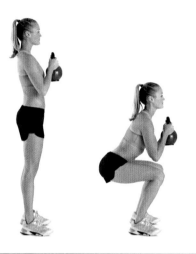

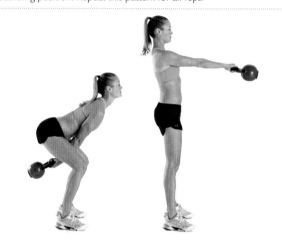

KETTLEBELL BURPEE

➡ Holding a pair of kettlebells, stand with your feet shoulder-width apart and your arms at your sides. Push your hips back, bend your knees, and lower your body as deeply as you can into a squat. Kick your legs backward, so that you're now in a pushup position. Perform a pushup on the kettlebells, then quickly bring your legs back to the squat position. Stand up quickly.

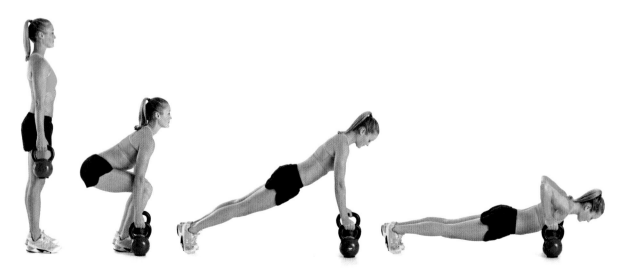

KETTLEBELL SINGLE-LEG ROMANIAN DEADLIFT

➡ Hold a pair of kettlebells in front of you with your knees slightly bent. Stand on your left leg and, keeping your back perfectly straight, hinge forward at your hips and lower the kettlebells to the ground. Your right leg will extend behind you. Pause, then return to the starting position. Repeat for the desired reps, then switch legs.

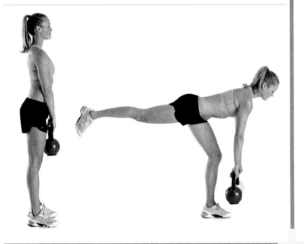

KETTLEBELL DOUBLE-LEG ROMANIAN DEADLIFT

➡ Hold a pair of kettlebells at arm's length in front of you, with your knees slightly bent. Without changing the bend in your knees, bend at your hips and lower your torso until it's almost parallel to the floor. Pause, then raise your torso to the starting position.

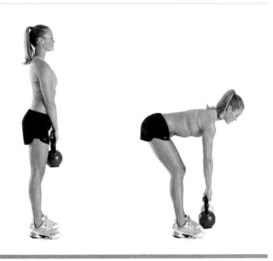

KETTLEBELL SINGLE-LEG ROMANIAN DEADLIFT (CONTRALATERAL)

➡ Hold a kettlebell in your right hand. Stand on your left leg, knee slightly bent, and, keeping your back perfectly straight, hinge forward at your hips and lower the kettlebell to the ground. Your right leg will extend behind you. Pause, then return to the starting position. Repeat for the desired reps, then switch, with the kettlebell in your left hand as you stand on your right leg.

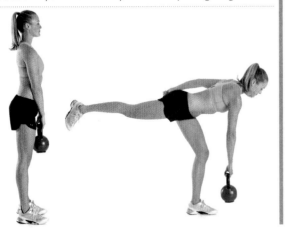

KETTLEBELL SINGLE-LEG ROMANIAN DEADLIFT (IPSILATERAL)

➡ Hold a kettlebell in your left hand. Stand on your left leg, knee slightly bent, and, keeping your back perfectly straight, hinge forward at your hips and lower the kettlebell to the ground. Your right leg will extend behind you. Pause, then return to the starting position. Repeat for the desired reps, then switch, with the kettlebell in your right hand as you stand on your right leg.

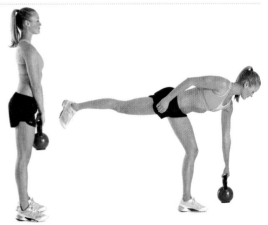

KETTLEBELL SUMO SQUAT

▶ Hold a kettlebell at arm's length in front of your thighs. Set your feet slightly wider than shoulder width, your toes turned slightly outward. Brace your abs, and lower your hips as far as you can by bending your knees and pushing your hips back. Keeping your hips back and your posture upright, explode to a standing position.

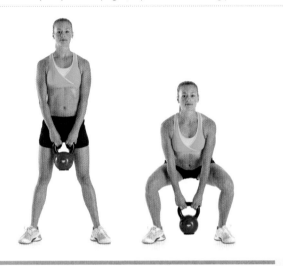

KETTLEBELL ALTERNATING HAMMER CURL

▶ Grab a pair of kettlebells and let them hang at arm's length next to your sides with your palms facing each other. Without moving your upper arms, bend your right elbow and curl one kettlebell up in front of your shoulder. As you lower the weight to the starting position, repeat with your left arm. That's 1 rep.

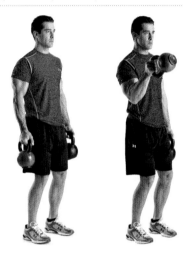

TRX LUNGE FULL LENGTH

▶ Face away from the anchor point, and place your right foot in both foot cradles of a TRX. Stand in a staggered stance. Lower your body until your right knee almost touches the floor and your left leg is bent 90 degrees. Press through your left heel to stand back up. Perform all your reps, then switch legs and repeat.

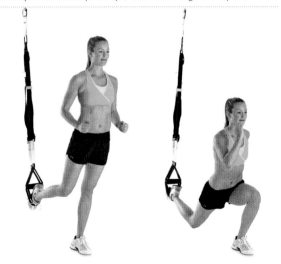

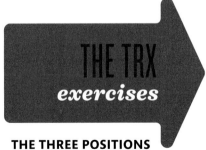

THE TRX
exercises

THE THREE POSITIONS OF THE TRX:

1. Full length (mid-calf level)

2. Mid length

3. Fully shortened

TRX BURPEE FULL LENGTH

➡ Place your right foot in both foot cradles of a TRX. Stand up tall on your left foot. Squat toward the floor by pushing your hips back and bending your left knee. Kick your legs back so you're in a pushup position with your body forming a straight line from your ankles to your neck. Perform a pushup, then bring your knees toward your chest, explode up on one leg, and jump. Return to the starting position. Do all your reps on your left leg, then switch legs and repeat.

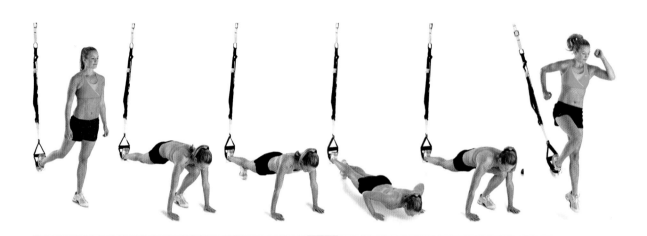

TRX JACKKNIFE AND PLANK FULL LENGTH

➡ Place both feet in the foot cradles of a TRX. Get into pushup position. Without moving your arms, bring your feet toward your waist and push your hips up. Your body should form an inverted V, with your back flat and your head between your arms. Pause and return to the starting position.

TRX PLANK FULL LENGTH

➡ Place both feet into the foot cradles of a TRX. Get into pushup position, your body forming a straight line from your ankles to your neck. Bend your elbows and lower your weight onto your forearms instead of your hands. Your elbows should be directly under your shoulders. Hold this position for the desired time, keeping your body stable and preventing your hips from sagging.

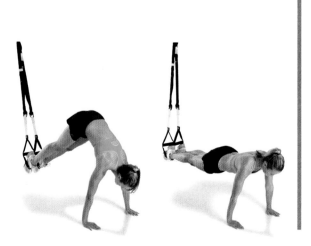

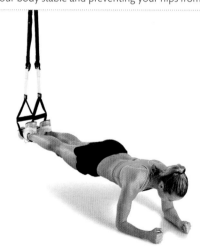

TRX ATOMIC PUSHUP FULL LENGTH

➡ Place both feet in the foot cradles of a TRX. Get into pushup position. Perform a pushup by lowering your body until your chest is just above the floor and then pressing back up. Bring your knees toward your elbows in a crunching movement. Pause and return to the starting position.

TRX ROW FULL LENGTH

➡ Hold onto the TRX and back away until you feel tension in the straps. Your body should form a 45- to 60-degree angle to the floor, and your arms should be parallel to the floor, palms down. Pull your body toward the anchor point by bringing the handles toward the sides of your chest as you rotate your palms inward. Your elbows should be at 45 degrees. Pause and return to the starting position.

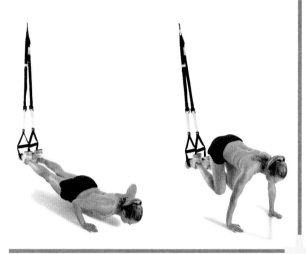

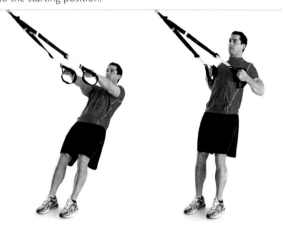

TRX JACKKNIFE AND PUSHUP FULL LENGTH

➡ Slide your feet into TRX foot cradles and get into pushup position. Perform a pushup, then slowly jackknife your body, raising your rear end as high as possible, while keeping your back and legs straight. Return to the starting position and repeat for the desired reps.

TRX TRICEPS EXTENSION MID LENGTH

➡ Face away from the anchor point of a TRX. Hold onto the TRX, extend your arms so they're at eye level, and walk away from the anchor until you feel tension in the straps. You should be leaning forward. Without changing the angle of your upper arms, bend your elbows until your hands are behind your head. Press back to the starting position by driving your hands forward until your arms are straight.

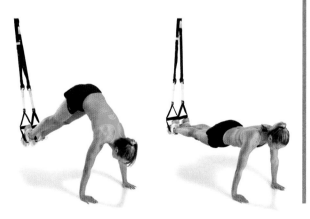

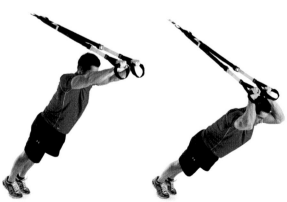

TRX CHEST PRESS   FULL LENGTH

➡ Face away from the anchor point of a TRX. Hold the handles in front of your chest with your arms extended. Your feet should be under the anchor point, and your arms high enough so the TRX does not rub your arms or shoulders. Lower your chest toward the handles until your hands are near your shoulders. Press back to the starting position.

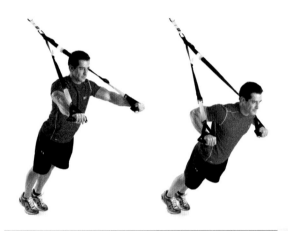

TRX T DELTOID FLY   FULL LENGTH

➡ Hold onto a TRX and back away until you feel tension in the straps. Your body should form a 45- to 60-degree angle to the floor, and your arms should be parallel to the floor. Pull your body toward the anchor point by pulling your hands away from each other and squeezing your shoulders together. When your arms are extended out, your body and arms should form a T. Return to the starting position.

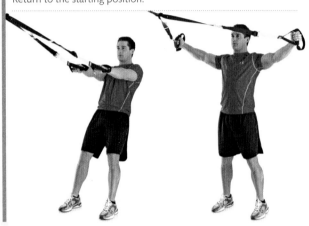

TRX I DELTOID FLY   FULL LENGTH

➡ Hold onto a TRX and back away until you feel tension in the straps. Your body should form a 45-degree angle to the floor, and your palms should be facing down. Raise your arms directly overhead, squeezing your shoulder blades together. Your body and arms should form an I. Return to the starting position.

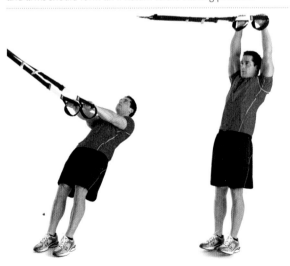

TRX Y DELTOID FLY   FULL LENGTH

➡ Hold onto a TRX and back away until you feel tension in the straps. Your body should form a 45- to 60-degree angle to the floor, and your palms should be facing down. Raise your arms overhead and to the sides at a 45-degree angle to your shoulders. Squeeze your shoulder blades together, and hold. Your body and arms should form a Y. Return to the starting position.

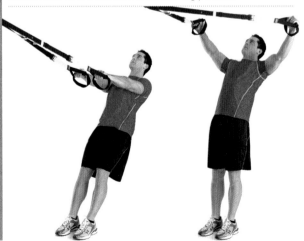

TRX PENDULUM SWING WITH KNEE TUCK
FULL LENGTH

▶ Slide your feet into TRX foot cradles and get into pushup position. Rotate your hips to the right and bring your knees toward your chest and outside the right shoulder. Swing your knees back through the middle, then repeat on your left side. Each tuck counts as 1 rep.

TRX BICEPS CURL   MID LENGTH

▶ Hold on to a TRX and back away until you feel tension in the straps. Your body should form a 45- to 60-degree angle to the floor, and your arms should be parallel to the floor, palms up. Without moving your upper arms, bend your elbows and curl the handles toward your shoulder, your palms facing your forehead. Pause and return to the starting position.

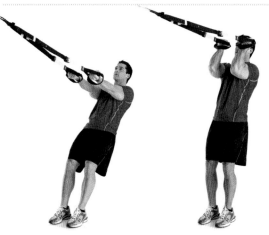

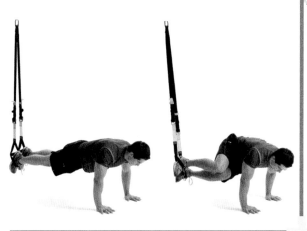

THE DUMBBELL *exercises*

DUMBBELL BICEPS CURL

▶ Grab a pair of dumbbells and let them hang at arm's length next to your sides, your palms facing each other. Without moving your upper arms, bend your elbows and raise the dumbbells as close to your shoulders as you can. As you lift the weights, rotate your palms so that they're facing up in the top position. Pause, then reverse the motion to return to the starting position.

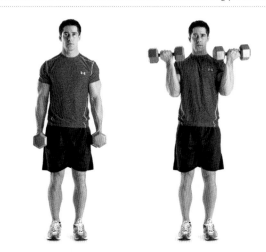

DUMBBELL ALTERNATING SHOULDER RAISE

➡ Holding a pair of dumbbells, rest your left hand in front of your left thigh with your palm facing down and your right arm to the side of your right thigh with your palm facing inward. With elbows slightly flexed, raise your right arm straight out to your side as you lift your left arm in front of you. When both arms are at shoulder level, pause, and then lower back to the starting position. Repeat for desired reps, then switch sides.

DUMBBELL ALTERNATING BICEPS CURL

➡ Grab a pair of dumbbells and let them hang at arm's length next to your sides, your palms facing each other. Without moving your upper arm, bend your elbow and curl one dumbbell as close to your shoulder as you can, while rotating your wrist so your palms face your body. Pause, then slowly lower the weight back to the starting position. Repeat on the other side.

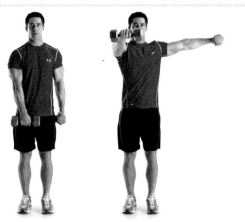

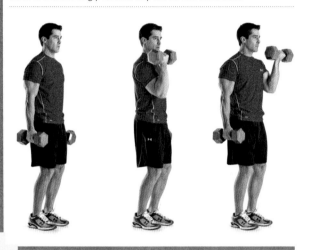

RENEGADE ROW

➡ Place a pair of dumbbells at the spots where you'd position your hands to do a pushup. Grasp the dumbbells and get into pushup position. Lower your body toward the floor, pause, then push yourself back up. Once you're back in the starting position, lift the dumbbell in your right hand to the right side of your chest. Lower the dumbbell back down, and repeat with your left arm. That's 1 rep.

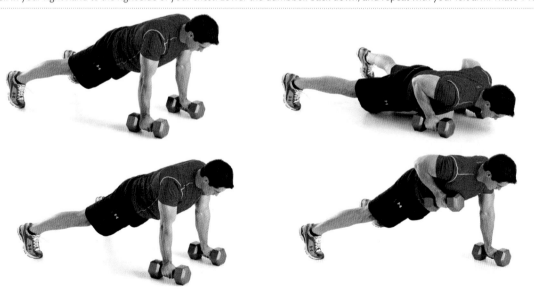

DUMBBELL CLEAN

➧ Hold a pair of dumbbells with an overhand grip while in a squat with your feet shoulder-width apart. In one movement, explosively lift the dumbbells as you straighten your hips and knees. When the dumbbells are at shoulder height, drop your hips and rotate your elbows so that the heads of the dumbbells face your shoulders. Rotate your elbows back so the dumbbells are in front of your chest, and lower your body to the starting position.

DUMBBELL CLEAN AND PRESS

➧ Hold a pair of dumbbells with an overhand grip while in a squat with your feet shoulder-width apart. In one movement, explosively lift the dumbbells as you straighten your hips and knees. When the dumbbells are at shoulder height, drop your hips and rotate your elbows so that the heads of the dumbbells face your shoulders. Then extend your arms up and press the dumbbells above your head. Lower the weights to the starting position.

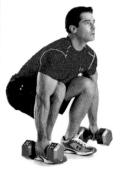

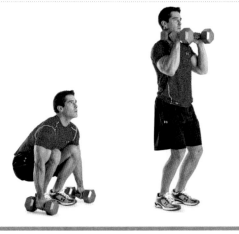

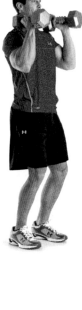

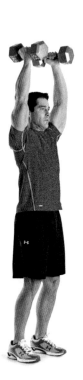

DUMBBELL POWER SHRUG

➧ Grab a pair of dumbbells and hold them at hip height. Stand with your feet shoulder-width apart. In one movement, thrust your hips forward, shrug your shoulders forcefully, and rise up onto your toes. Lower yourself back down onto your heels.

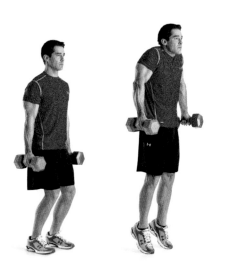

DUMBBELL HITCHHIKER

➡ Hold a light dumbbell in your left hand and extend it overhead so that your elbow is bent 90 degrees and your left arm is perpendicular to your body. With your palm facing away from your body, bring your left hand down and across your body so that your left thumb ends up near your right pants pocket. Extend your left arm back up and away and finish with your thumb facing up and away at the top. Do the desired reps, then switch sides.

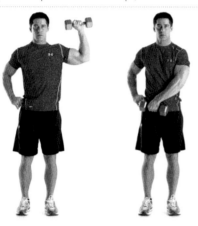

DUMBBELL SINGLE-ARM SCARECROW

➡ Grab a dumbbell in your right hand and raise your upper arm so it is parallel to the floor. Your palms should be facing away from your body with your elbows bent at 90 degrees. Without changing the position of your upper arm, rotate your right forearm up and back as far as you can. Hold for a moment, and then return to the starting position. Do all the reps with your right arm, then repeat with your left.

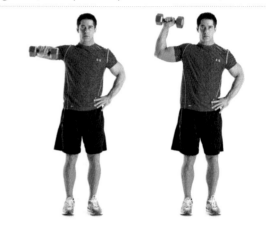

DUMBBELL DOUBLE-ARM SCARECROW

➡ Hold a dumbbell in each hand and raise your upper arms so that they're parallel to the floor. Without changing the position of your upper arms, internally rotate your forearms down as far as possible. Then switch directions and externally rotate your forearms back as far as possible. Return to the starting position.

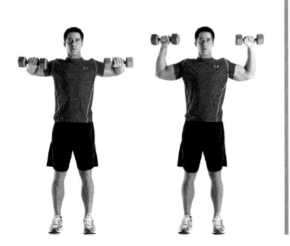

DUMBBELL WALKING LUNGE

➡ Hold a pair of dumbbells at arm's length next to your sides, your palms facing each other. Step forward with your left leg and slowly lower your body until your knee is bent at least 90 degrees. Pause, then push yourself to the starting position as quickly as you can. Complete the prescribed number of reps with your left leg, then repeat with your right leg.

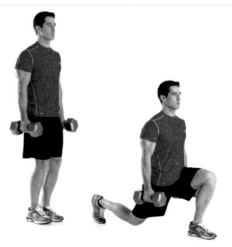

DEATH CRAWL

➡ Place a pair of dumbbells at the spots where you position your hands for a pushup. Grasp the dumbbells and get into pushup position. Lower your body to the floor, pause, then push yourself back up. Once you're back in the starting position, lift the dumbbell in your right hand to the right side of your chest. Lower the dumbbell back down and repeat with your left arm. Then "walk" each hand one step forward and follow with your feet so you're back in the starting position. That's 1 rep.

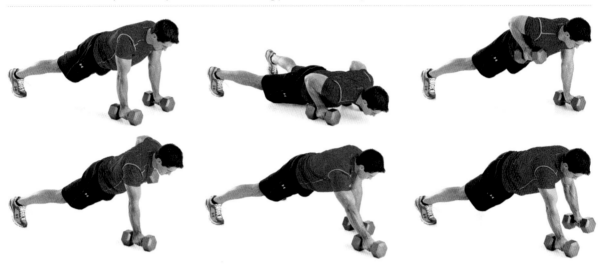

DUMBBELL SIDE LUNGE

➡ Hold a dumbbell in your right hand at arm's length, your palm facing your body. Lift your left foot and take a big step to your left as you push your hips backward and lower your body by dropping your hips and bending your left knee. Your right leg should remain straight, and your right arm should hang in front of you. Pause, then return to the starting position.

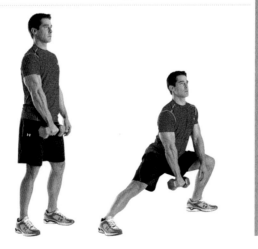

DUMBBELL SINGLE-ARM ROW

➡ Grab a dumbbell in your left hand and place your right hand and right knee on a flat bench. Your lower back should be naturally arched and your torso roughly parallel to the floor. Keeping your upper arm perpendicular to your body, row the weight toward the side of your chest. Pause, and then return to the starting position. Complete all your reps, then switch sides and repeat.

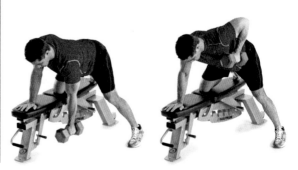

BICEPS 10/10/10

▶ Grab a pair of dumbbells and let them hang at arm's length next to your sides, your palms facing inward. Raise your left forearm so your elbow is bent 90 degrees, rotate the palm upward, and hold it there. Perform a set of 10 dumbbell curls with your right arm. After you've finished all your reps with your right arm, switch arms, performing the static hold with your right arm and curling 10 times with your left. Then perform simultaneous curls with both arms for 1 more set of 10 reps.

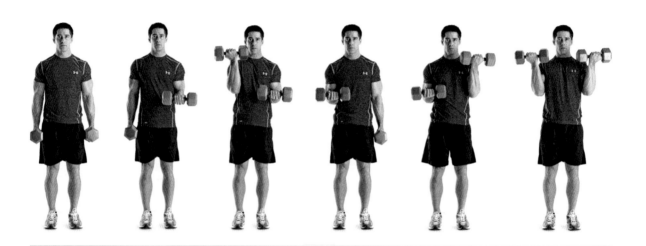

DUMBBELL BENCH PRESS

▶ Grab a pair of dumbbells and lie on your back on a flat bench, holding the dumbbells over your chest so that they're nearly touching, your palms facing forward. Lower the weights to the sides of your chest, rotating your wrists so that your palms face each other. Pause, then press the weights back up to the starting position.

DUMBBELL ALTERNATING BENCH PRESS

▶ Grab a pair of dumbbells, lie on your back on a flat bench, and hold the dumbbells above your chest. Your palms should be facing forward. Lower one dumbbell to the side of your chest, while simultaneously rotating your wrists so your palm faces inward. Pause, then press the weight back up to the starting position as fast as possible, as you rotate your wrists so your palms are once again facing forward. Repeat with the other arm.

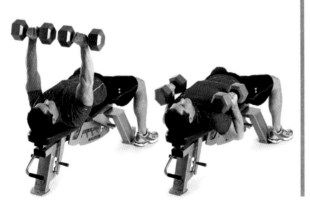

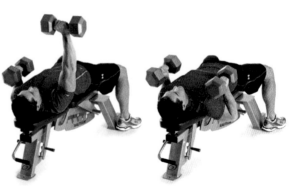

DUMBBELL INCLINE ALTERNATING BENCH PRESS

➡ Set an adjustable bench to about a 30-degree angle. Lie faceup on the bench and hold the dumbbells above your shoulders with your arms straight and palms facing forward. Lower one dumbbell to your chest and twist the dumbbell so your palms face each other. Pause, then press the weight back up to the starting position, and repeat with your other arm. That's 1 rep.

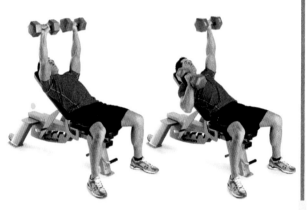

DUMBBELL INCLINE BENCH PRESS

➡ Set an adjustable bench to about a 30-degree incline. Lie faceup on the bench and hold a pair of dumbbells above your shoulders with your arms straight, palms facing forward. Lower the weights to your chest and twist your wrists so your palms face each other. Pause, then press the weights back up to the starting position as fast as possible, as you rotate your wrists so your palms are once again facing forward.

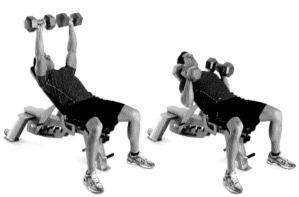

DUMBBELL SINGLE-ARM INCLINE BENCH PRESS

➡ Grab one dumbbell and lie faceup on a bench. Hold the dumbbell above your chest with your arm straight and palm facing forward, and extend your other arm out to the side, perpendicular to your torso. Lower the dumbbell to your chest and twist the dumbbell so your palm faces your body. Pause, then press the weight back up to the starting position. Complete all reps, switch arms, and repeat.

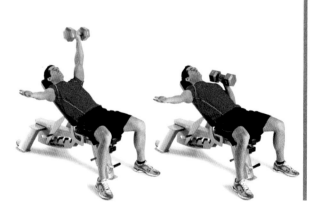

ROLLING TRICEPS SUPERSET

➡ Grab a pair of dumbbells and lie faceup on a bench with the dumbbells resting near your armpits. Without changing the angle of your elbows, lower the dumbbells behind your head. Pause, then raise the dumbbells back to the starting position. Then press the dumbbells straight above your chest until your arms are extended. That's 1 rep.

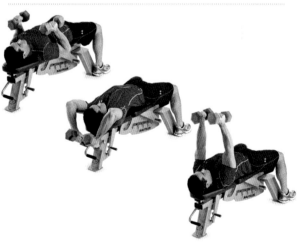

DUMBBELL FLOOR PRESS

➡ Grab a pair of dumbbells and lie faceup on the floor. Rest your upper arms on the floor with your palms facing inward. Press the weights up above your chest and turn your hands so that your palms face forward. Slowly return to the starting position.

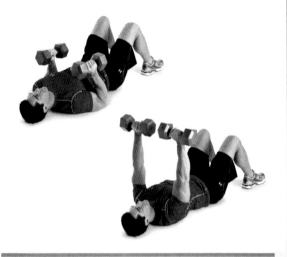

DUMBBELL STEPDOWN

➡ Stand on your left leg on a bench or box that's about knee height. Hold a pair of dumbbells at arm's length at your sides (or straight out in front of your chest). Balancing on your left foot, bend your left knee and slowly lower your body until your right heel lightly touches the floor. Pause, then lift yourself back up with your left leg. Do all your reps with your left leg, then repeat with your right.

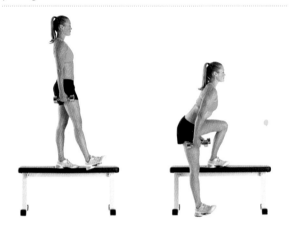

DUMBBELL STEPUP

➡ Hold a pair of dumbbells at arm's length at your sides. Stand facing a bench that's about knee height. Step up onto the bench with your right leg, and then step up onto the bench with your left leg. Return to the starting position by stepping down with your right leg first and then the left. Repeat for the desired reps, then switch legs.

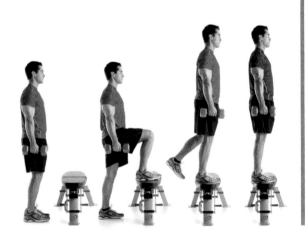

LAT PULLDOWN

➡ Sit at a lat pulldown station and grab the bar with an overhand grip that's just beyond shoulder width. Your arms should be completely straight and above your chest. Without moving your torso, pull the bar down to your chest by squeezing your shoulder blades. Pause, then return to the starting position.

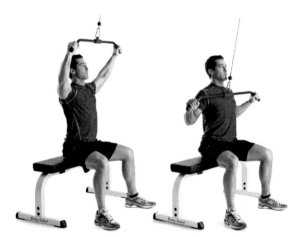

OVERHEAD LUNGE

➥ Stand holding a barbell in an overhead grip. Press the barbell overhead. Step forward with your left leg and lower your body until your knee is bent at least 90 degrees. Pause, then push yourself to the starting position as quickly as you can. Repeat the movement, this time stepping forward with your right leg. Continue to alternate legs.

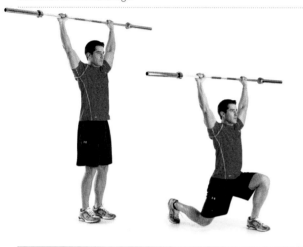

BUS DRIVER

➥ Wrap a towel around one end of a barbell and wedge that end firmly into a bench. Grab the other end with both hands and hold it in front of your left hip. Your right (back) foot should rotate inward. In a sweeping arc (while keeping your arms straight), twist your torso to bring the barbell in front of your body. Finish with the barbell in the other direction. (Twist your right foot a bit as the bar moves across your body.) Repeat in the other direction.

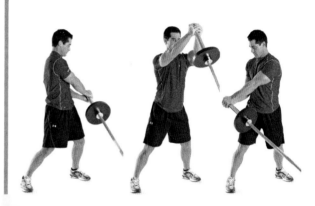

BUS DRIVER ROTATIONAL DROP STEP

➥ Wedge one end of a barbell into a bench as in the bus driver. Squat and grab the other end with your left hand, with your arm fully extended. Step back with your right foot and pull the barbell up to your rib cage as you stand and rotate your body so you face the barbell, finishing with the bar at shoulder height. Return to the starting position. Do all your left-arm reps, then switch sides, and repeat.

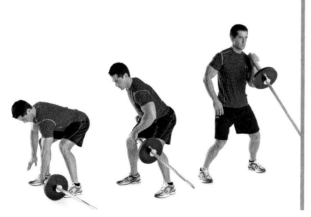

BUS DRIVER SQUAT PRESS

➥ Wedge one end of a barbell into a bench as in the bus driver. Squat and hold the other end in your right hand. Stand and push the barbell until your arm is extended. Return to the starting position. Do all your reps with your right arm, then repeat with your left.

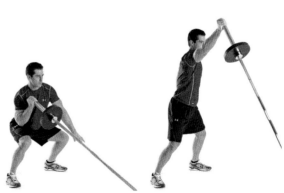

BARBELL BENCH PRESS

➡ Grasp a barbell with an overhand grip that's just wider than shoulder width and hold it above your torso with your arms completely straight. Lower the bar down toward your sternum, pause, then press the bar back up to the starting position.

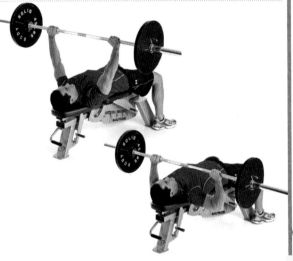

BARBELL DEADLIFT

➡ Load a barbell and roll it against your shins. Bend at your hips and knees and grab the bar with an overhand grip or a mixed grip, your hands just beyond shoulder width. Without allowing your lower back to round, pull your torso back and up, thrust your hips forward, and stand up with the barbell. Lower the bar to the floor, keeping it as close to your body as possible.

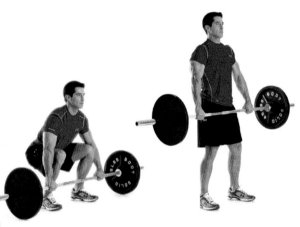

SUPERBAND CHEST STRETCH

➡ Grab a Superband with your hands about 2 feet apart. Stand tall with your feet shoulder-width apart and raise the Superband above your head. Then pull the Superband behind your head to stretch your chest. Hold for the desired time.

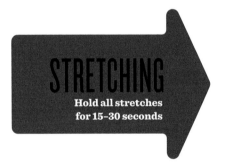

STRETCHING
**Hold all stretches
for 15–30 seconds**

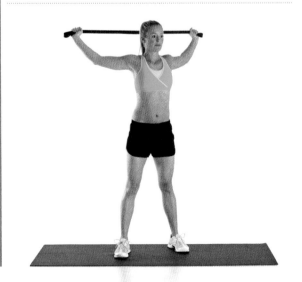

KNEELING HIP FLEXOR STRETCH

➡ Kneel on your left knee with your right knee upright. Keeping your chest up, push your hips forward and stretch your left arm above your head. Hold for the desired time.

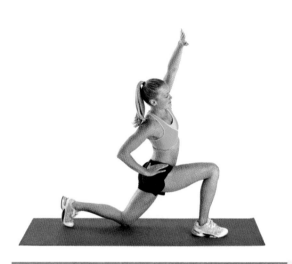

CAT AND DOG

➡ Position yourself on your hands and knees. Gently arch your midback and simultaneously tuck your chin toward your chest. Then switch the direction and arch your lower back as you look up toward the ceiling. Slowly alternate between these positions.

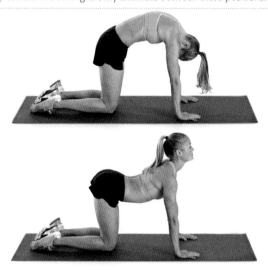

DOWNWARD DOG

➡ Start in pushup position. Sink your heels toward the floor and press your chest back toward your thighs. Hold for desired time.

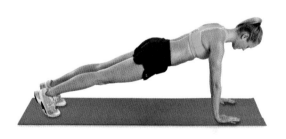

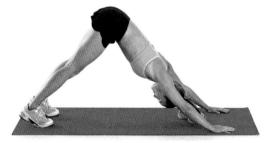

UPWARD DOG

➡ Start in pushup position, and then roll forward over your toes without letting your thighs touch the floor. Keep your upper legs off the floor and drop your hips. Make sure your shoulders stay over your wrists and your chest stretches upward. Hold for the desired time.

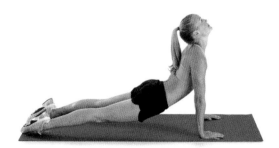

PIGEON POSE

➡ Get down on all fours on the floor, with your wrists under your shoulders and your knees under your hips. As you extend your left leg back, bend your right knee and invert your right leg forward so it's in front of your left leg. Bend your torso over your right leg so the weight of your body rests on your right leg.

FIGURE-4 STRETCH

➡ Lying on your back, invert your leg so your right foot rests on your left knee. Place both hands behind your left leg, and pull it toward your chest until you feel a stretch in your right hip and glute. Hold it for 30 seconds, then switch sides.

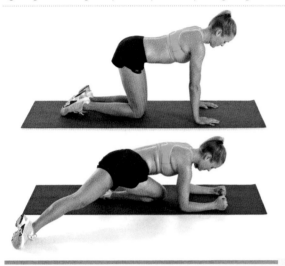

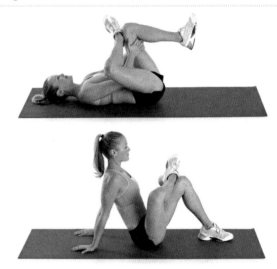

SUPERBAND HAMSTRING STRETCH

➡ Lie on your back, wrap a Superband around the bottom of your right foot, and grasp the other side of the band. Keeping your right leg as straight as possible, lift it up in the air and stretch your right hamstring. Your left leg should remain flat on the floor throughout the stretch. Hold for the desired time, then switch legs and repeat.

SUPERBAND GROIN STRETCH

➡ Lie on your back, wrap a Superband around the bottom of your left foot, and grasp the other side of the band. Keep your left leg straight, and lift it to the side as far as possible. Your right leg should remain flat on the ground throughout the stretch. Hold for the desired time, then switch legs and repeat.

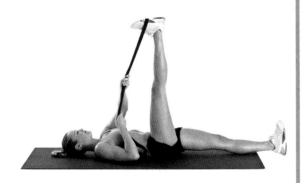

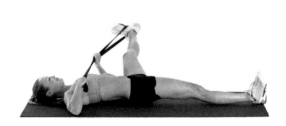

SUPERBAND LOWER-BACK STRETCH

▶ Lie on your back, wrap a Superband around the bottom of your right foot, and grasp the other side of the band. Keeping your right leg as straight as possible, lift your right leg over your left leg and as far over to the left as you can. Your left leg should remain flat on the floor throughout the stretch. Hold for the desired time, then switch legs and repeat.

SUPERBAND SIDE-LYING QUAD/HIP FLEXOR

▶ Lie on your back, wrap a Superband around the bottom of your left foot, and grasp the other side of the band. Roll over onto your right side so that the Superband is behind your head and your left knee is flexed behind you. Your right leg should remain flat on the floor throughout the stretch. Hold for the desired time, then switch legs and repeat.

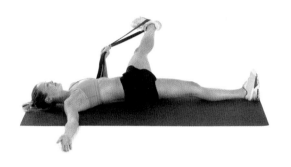

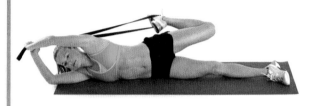

IMPACT! Alternative Exercise List

All exercises in this book are ones that I feel give you the most bang for your buck. They are real, authentic movements that I use every day at my facility, Fitness Quest 10. But the movements are not limited to the equipment found in this book. While I believe that these simple, yet highly effective tools are the best way to train your body and see results, I never want a piece of equipment to be an excuse for why you aren't training. If you don't have a TRX or Superbands, you can use these exercise alternatives.

THE EXERCISE	THE REPLACEMENT
TRX ROW	RACK ROW OR DB SINGLE-ARM ROW
TRX BICEPS CURL	DB CURL
TRX SUSPENDED LUNGE	BOSU BULGARIAN LUNGE
TRX BURPEE	KB BURPEE
TRX ATOMIC PUSHUP	BOSU BURPEE
TRX PLANK	PLANK
TRX I, Y, AND T DELTOID FLY	SC I, Y, AND T DELTOID FLY
TRX CHEST PRESS	BOSU PUSHUP
TRX TRICEPS EXTENSION	SC TRICEPS EXTENSION
SB CHOP (HIGH TO LOW)	SC CHOP (HIGH TO LOW)
SB LIFT (LOW TO HIGH)	SC CHOP (LOW TO HIGH)
½-KNEELING SB CHOP	½-KNEELING SC CHOP
½-KNEELING SB LIFT	½-KNEELING SC LIFT
SB ROTATION	SC ROTATION
SB LATERAL BAND WALK	SC LATERAL WALK
SB UPRIGHT ROW	SC UPRIGHT ROW
SB BICEPS CURL	SC BICEPS CURL
SB SQUAT AND SINGLE-ARM ROW AND ROTATE	SC SQUAT AND SINGLE-ARM ROW AND ROTATE
SB SINGLE-ARM ½-KNEELING PULLDOWN	SC SINGLE-ARM PULLDOWN
SB SEATED PULLDOWN	LAT PULLDOWN
SC HITCHHIKER	DB HITCHHIKER
SC SINGLE-ARM SCARECROW	DB SINGLE-ARM SCARECROW
SC DOUBLE-ARM SCARECROW	DB DOUBLE-ARM SCARECROW

appendix
FITNESS ON THE GO

 "Time is like money; the less we have of it to spare, the further we make it go."

—JOSH BILLINGS

I'm a road warrior. I take more than 30 business trips a year, and let me tell you, I know how hard it is to maintain your exercise and eating program while on the road. It's crazy: You're distracted by travel demands, different time zones, unfamiliar surroundings, and, of course, planes, trains, and automobiles, which seem designed to suck the energy out of you by the time you arrive at your destination.

Guess what: None of that is an excuse to miss your workouts or trash good eating habits. You know me, I love eliminating excuses. If traveling or a packed schedule makes it harder to stay on the program, then this chapter exists to make it easier. I've learned a lot about maximizing limited time and tools on my road trips—and it's all in this chapter.

Here you'll find a variety of 10-minute and 20-minute "body blaster" workouts you can do anytime, anywhere. It doesn't matter if you're on the road or just want to squeeze in a quick workout during your busy day.

I've also packed this chapter full of tips for smart traveling, whether you're flying cross-country or trapped in your car for hours. Follow my advice and you'll feel great when you get where you're going.

Fitness on the go: It's not an option; it's a necessity.

IMPACT Tips
for High-Performance Traveling

▶ **1. PREPARE!** With both your eating and your exercise, you must pack for success. I always bring my Superband and TRX if I'm traveling for more than 2 days. Both items pack easily and travel well. Between body weight and my "traveling gym," I know I'll never skip a workout when on the road. I also pack food. (See "Eat Great on the Go.")

▶ **2. ELIMINATE EXCUSES.** Stop sabotaging yourself by skipping workouts on the road because of the two biggest excuses out there:

"I don't have time!"
"I don't have a gym on the road!"

Everyone uses the first excuse—they're busy in meetings, they have social events to attend, they've got itineraries to maintain, and the excuses go on and on. "I don't have time." Boy, that really lets you off the hook, doesn't it? It's perfect. Well, forget it, because it no longer exists.

We all have time for our priorities, and you need to start prioritizing your health and fitness in any situation. Get up early in your "new" city, get in "only" a 20-minute workout (there are two great ones in this chapter), walk to your meeting instead of taking a taxi, or cut down on the socializing on the business trip to ensure you're getting in your full workouts.

That second excuse is popular with folks who think they need a first-class facility to get in a great workout when on the road. Don't get me wrong— a great gym is a terrific motivator. I actually choose to stay at hotels that I know have good fitness facilities with free weights. I supply the TRX and Superband, and I get an all-out sweat.

But if you're stuck in a hotel with the dreaded "fitness center" with one treadmill and a TV? Use the workouts in this chapter, naturally, but how about also just going outside and doing some great

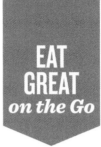

EAT GREAT on the Go

▶ **DRINK UP.** Carry a liter of water with you at all times. Especially on airplanes. The dry cabin air dehydrates you, especially if you're flying for more than a couple of hours. Remember, drink half your body weight in fluid ounces of water daily.

▶ **PACK SMART SNACKS.** I never go anywhere without good food—the kind of food that makes it easy to ignore the unhealthy options available on the road or in airports. Some examples:
•Protein bars
•Trail mix
•Fresh fruit that travels well (apple, pear, banana)
•Precut raw veggies
•Tuna or sardines
•Bag of prepackaged almonds

▶ **EAT FOR THE NEW TIME ZONE.** Do your best to time your meals to correspond with the local time so you can maintain a normal eating schedule.

▶ **LEARN HOW TO MANAGE MEALS AWAY FROM HOME.** Remember that you select what you eat and when. Use these tips on your next trip. The hotel breakfast bar has everything you need to start the day right: fruit, oatmeal, and omelets. Focus on lots of veggies. Ask for egg whites only. At lunch and dinner, try ordering without a menu. And what about the dreaded conference buffets? Do what I do: Focus on fruit, greens, a whole grain roll, and the carving station for a lean protein. Done.

▶ **MIND YOUR ALCOHOL CONSUMPTION.** Travel is tough on your body. One way to make it easier is to reduce or eliminate alcohol from your travel diet. It's dehydrating, can interrupt your sleep, and provides nothing but empty calories. Alcohol will never be the "and then some" that's good for you.

▶ **FIND A LOCAL GROCERY STORE.** When you reach your destination, load up on healthy choices that you can store in your room (water, fruit, nuts, and protein bars).

cardio as you take a city tour on foot? It gets you outside, changes your environment, and is good for your mind. Looking for more? Throw your TRX and Superband in a backpack and set out for a little adventure. You can wrap your TRX around a light pole or tree branch (pick one that won't break) and bang out a nice 5- to 10-minute TRX routine at random spots! This all is about play!

IMPACT Workouts
on the Go!

The workouts break down like this:

▶ Two different 10-minute body-weight workouts. One is basic, the second a bit more intense. You don't need any equipment to do them. I like them because they are time efficient, work the entire body, and involve conditioning. They will certainly leave you feeling breathless, as your rest times will be short and your tempo will be quick. Just fire it up and get after it!

▶ A TRX travel workout. That's the beauty of the TRX. It takes up very little space in your carry-on luggage, so you have no excuse not to bring it with you on every trip. And your TRX comes with a door anchor that's as stable as any pullup bar you'll find at the gym. (With some TRX sets, this door anchor is sold separately.) It truly is like carrying a gym with you wherever you go.

> *"Most people give up just when they're about to achieve success. They quit on the 1 yard line. They give up in the last minute of the game, 1 foot from a winning touchdown."*
>
> — H. ROSS PEROT

Get Ready to Sweat /// Don't think these workouts using the Superband or TRX will be challenging? Try again. These are staples of my program at Fitness Quest 10, and it's really no different from what you would do in the gym. You can work your entire body, improve your conditioning, and have some serious fun with these simple yet highly effective, travel-friendly pieces of equipment.

A Superband travel workout. A Superband is even easier to travel with than a TRX—after all, it's just a big rubber band. Twenty minutes in your hotel room and you're done!

A body-weight travel workout. No TRX or Superbands? No problem. This body-weight workout will take you to the edge of your endurance. You'll love it—and be finished in 20 minutes.

These workouts are difference makers. Using them—or not using them—will be the difference for a lot of people between true success on the IMPACT program and mediocre performance. It's that simple.

I've eliminated every possible excuse for you. Now, as always, it comes down to action. 10 in—10 out. Don't let lack of time or lack of facilities stop you from having an amazing workout! Those two excuses create your biggest moments of weakness and temptation: "Hmmm, I'm really busy today, I'm on the road, maybe I'll just skip the workout today. No big deal."

It is a big deal. You're allowing the little voice in your head to run your life. When was the last time that worked out well for you?

Come on, get it done. Read your IMPACT card, put on some great tunes, fire yourself up, and blast your body! No more excuses! 10 in—10 out, and then some, baby!

> ## "The true measure of a man is not how he behaves in moments of comfort and convenience but how he stands at times of controversy and challenge."
>
> —MARTIN LUTHER KING JR.

An Important Message /// These workouts should be used only when you absolutely, positively are short on time and facilities. They are very effective, but they are also the exception, not the rule. The IMPACT program is designed for full workouts. These shorter workouts will do in a pinch, but they are not a substitute for your normal, complete workout. Remember: 10 in—10 out! No shortcuts!

10-Minute Body-Weight Express
Workout A
BEGINNER

1
LUNGE
STRAIGHT, DIAGONAL, AND/OR SIDE

➡ 3 x 20 | pp. 222, 233

PUSHUP

➡ 3 x max | p. 229

2
STAR JUMP

➡ 2 x 10 | p. 227

BICYCLE AND ROTATE

➡ 2 x max | p. 228

3
WALK, JOG, OR RUN INTERVALS

➡ 5 sets of 30 seconds on, 30 seconds off

10-Minute Body-Weight Express
Workout B
INTERMEDIATE

1
SQUAT JUMP

➡ 1 x 10 | p. 234

2
PUSHUP

➡ 1 x max | p. 229

3
LUNGE HOP

➡ 1 x 20 | p. 233

4
PUSHUP

➡ 1 x max | p. 229

5
SKATER PLYO

➡ 1 x 20 | p. 230

Repeat circuit 2 times with minimal rest between exercises, and 90 seconds to 2 minutes off between circuit 1 and circuit 2.

GRAND FINALE
CONDITIONING
after workout

SPRINTS

1A. Sprint
1 minute
1B. Bicycle and rotate p. 228
Max reps

REST

2A. Sprint
30 seconds
2B. Hipup p. 231
20 reps / side

REST

3A. Sprint to fatigue
3B. Plank p. 228
Hold as long as possible.

TRX Travel Routine
20 minutes

1
TRX ROW
➡ 1 x 10–15 | p. 255

2
TRX BICEPS CURL
➡ 1 x 10–15 | p. 257

3
TRX CHEST PRESS
➡ 1 x 10–15 | p. 256

4
TRX TRICEPS EXTENSION
➡ 1 x 10–15 | p. 255

Repeat circuit 2 times.

5
TRX LUNGE
➡ 1 x 10–15 | p. 253

6
TRX JACKKNIFE AND PUSHUP
➡ 1 x 10–15 | p. 255

7
TRX PENDULUM SWING WITH KNEE TUCK
➡ 1 x 10–20 | p. 257

8
TRX PLANK
➡ 1 x 10–15 | p. 254

Do exercises 5, 6, 7, and 8 only 1 time.

Optional: Grand Finale Conditioning

Superband Travel Routine
20 minutes

1
SUPERBAND LATERAL WALK
➡ 2 x 15 | p. 243

SUPERBAND UPRIGHT ROW
➡ 2 x 15 | p. 243

2
SUPERBAND SQUAT AND SINGLE-ARM ROW AND ROTATE
➡ 2 x 10 / side | p. 247

SUPERBAND ROTATION
➡ 2 x 10 / side | p. 245

3
SUPERBAND SPLIT-SQUAT ANTIROTATION
➡ 2 x 10 | p. 244

SUPERBAND SPLITTER
➡ 2 x 10–15 | p. 242

4
SUPERBAND OVERHEAD TRICEPS EXTENSION/ PRESSDOWN
➡ 1 x max | p. 246

SUPERBAND HAMMER CURL
➡ 1 x max | p. 243

5
SUPERBAND RESISTED PUSHUP
➡ 1 x 20 | p. 247

SUPERBAND SEATED PULLDOWN
➡ 1 x max | p. 246

Optional: Grand Finale Conditioning

CONDITIONING
after workout

For TRX or Superband

Choose one:

1. 5 MINUTES "TEMPO"

Walk, jog, or run as fast as you can for 5 minutes.

2. SPRINTS

5 sets of 30 seconds on, 30 seconds off. If time permits, 5-10 minutes of cardio.

3. PLYOMETRIC ROUTINE

a. Squat jump p. 234
1 x 10
b. Lunge hop p. 233
1 x 20
c. Skater plyo p. 230
1 x 20
d. Pushup p. 229
1 x max

Repeat circuit 2 times, if time permits.

20-Minute Body-Weight Travel Routine

As little rest time as possible between exercises; 1-2 minutes between circuits; 1-2 minutes between stations.

WARMUP: Walk or jog for 5–10 minutes.

STATION 1

1
LUNGE

➡ 1 x 30 | p. 233

2
PUSHUP

➡ 1 x 20 | p. 229

3
SINGLE-LEG BALANCE TOUCH

➡ 1 x 10 / leg | p. 225

4
SPRINT

➡ 2 minutes

Repeat circuit 3 times.

STATION 2

5
DIRTY DOG

➡ 1 x 20 | p. 226

6
HORSEBACK RIDING

➡ 1 x 10 forward / 10 backward | p. 227

7
BIRD DOG AND ROTATE

➡ 1 x 10 / side | p. 226

8
PUSHUP

➡ 1 x 10 | p. 229

Repeat circuit 2 times, then run for 1 minute.

STATION 3

9
HELLO DOLLY

➡ 1 x 20 | p. 232

10
BICYCLE AND ROTATE

➡ Approximately 20 seconds | p. 228

11
HIPUP

➡ 1 x 20 / side | p. 231

12
SUPERMAN

➡ 1 x 20 | p. 233

Repeat circuit 2 times.

Do cardio for as much time as you have remaining.

Index

Boldface page references indicate photographs. <u>Underscored</u> references indicate boxed text, charts, and marginalia.